THE **EATING** *ENIGMA*

THE
EATING
ENIGMA

Unlocking the gates to a secret garden,
removing emotional weeds, and cultivating change.

MARIA AYNE, R.H.N.

Crown Oak Press

Crown Oak Press
2301 Lucien Way #415
Maitland, FL 32751
407.339.4217
www.crownoakpress.com

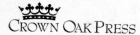

CROWN OAK PRESS

Printed in the United States of America.

Unless otherwise indicated, Scripture quotations taken from the Holy Bible, New International Version (NIV). Copyright © 1973, 1978, 1984, 2011 by Biblica, Inc.™. Used by permission. All rights reserved.

ISBN: 9781545616772

For my mother, Lisa.

Table of Contents

Introduction

Once upon a time, I used to eat ice cream for breakfast. Occasionally, if I managed to shove the first bowl down my throat fast enough (and before anyone in my family woke up to find me), I may have even "treated" myself to seconds. The disconcerting truth is that these were my eating patterns for the remainder of the day, week, month, and, before I knew it, the proceeding 20 years. To claim that I had a food addiction was an understatement, to say the least.

It's a bit of a difficult story to digest for anyone who knows me today. Presently, I'm a registered holistic nutritionist who is truly tickled at the sight of a salad. Throughout the years, I've abandoned everything that no longer served me, and have dedicated my life to not only understanding what causes eating disorders and what it takes to overcome emotional eating and food addictions, but to further cultivate a loving, harmonious relationship among mind, body, and food.

While I greatly encourage you to read this book in its entirety, if you want to gain any real insight into how I managed to do this, I will provide you with a short answer right here and now, so you can determine if this book is right for you. The short answer is: work. Lots and lots of work. Let me assure you, however, that not only is it well and truly possible, but the rewards outweigh the drawbacks by a hefty score.

While patience and dedication to my cause were key virtues on the journey, they alone were not enough. I needed to address several other critical factors if I wanted to unravel my emotional eating enigma. Regardless of the fact that I have included a few activities, it is important not to mistake this book for a how-to guide, as there's already a surplus of those kinds of publications in the world. Despite these beautifully written and informative guides, the statistics show that we are sicker and more obese than ever. I have the greatest respect for these books, as they do have their place, but that is not the intention here.

In all fairness, you already know how to eat spinach; you already know how to drive to the gym, and you likely already know how to do a sit-up or make a salad. There's no question that you also already know what *not* to do; the mere fact that you cringed at the idea of me admitting to eating ice cream for breakfast as a child should be regarded as a great insight that you have an intrinsic sense of what are and are not healthy choices.

Making the distinction between healthy habits and destructive habits is an innate ability we all share, but we have been conditioned since birth to ignore our intuition and to ultimately go against our natural instincts. We can all identify that a salad is healthy and a donut is unhealthy, but we can't always say that 100 percent of the time we choose the salad over the donut. When it comes to stimulants, such as junk food, we make the choice to "use" them, knowing that they are disastrous to the body, even though intentionally causing harm to ourselves goes against both our natural instincts and our evolutionary design.

For example, the thought of intentional bodily harm, such as slicing our own flesh or piercing our own skin with a needle, gives us a visceral reaction that makes it almost unbearable to imagine. Yet somehow, slow suicide through destructive lifestyle choices doesn't create the same effect. We all know the difference between real, wholesome food versus unhealthy, harmful food. Therefore, the struggle is not in the what, nor is it in the how, but rather in the why. My mission here is to educate you on the why, so you can arm yourself with your newfound knowledge to sort out your own eating enigma, and learn how to overcome it.

The objective of this book is to unveil the many masks of this compulsion and to provide you with a greater understanding of the force that you have granted the power to dominate your life. The intention is for you to become so familiar with this insidious habit that you can become the master, thus rendering it no longer useful in your world. After all, the only real way to gain control over anything in life is to first understand the mechanisms by which it works so that you can indeed overpower it.

Because this is not a how-to guide, it's best not to interpret the chapters as steps. The order in which the chapters are presented is not meant to reflect their hierarchy or the ideal sequence in which they should be examined. This book should also not be considered as a means to cure food addiction. Instead, I encourage you to think of it more as a little inspiration to push you in the right direction, and that path is completely dependent on your individual desires.

It is important to note that there is a distinction between those who simply find eating pleasurable—which is a normal and natural process—and those who have developed a hazardous relationship with food, such as binge eating and/or food addiction. There is an essential biochemical feedback loop that is governed by our hormones and neurochemicals that is responsible for the pleasurable feelings of eating. These powerful chemicals make it immensely satisfying to remedy hunger by seeking out food and further devouring each and every bite until we feel full and satiated.

Ghrelin, also known as the "hunger hormone," helps regulate appetite; when the stomach is empty, ghrelin is secreted and stimulates the production of the neurochemical dopamine. Dopamine spurs us to turn our attention toward the prospect of finding food and makes eating feel highly pleasurable. The hungrier we become, the harder it is to concentrate on any activity other than eating. Once we've eaten and the stomach lining begins to stretch, ghrelin secretion comes to a halt and an alternate hormone, leptin, is released instead. Leptin, "the satiety hormone," travels to our brain and signals us to stop eating, at which point our appetite begins to curb; our sense of taste starts to diminish, and we lose interest in food. Because leptin dulls the dopamine spike, the pleasurable sensation decreases and thus we no longer feel the desire to eat.

When something causes us to voraciously eat past this point, something has gone very wrong. Uncontrollable eating when we are no longer hungry is not a part of the natural phenomenon that ensures our survival, but rather a cataclysmic force that is overpowering people in staggering numbers.

Despite the rise in obesity, eating disorders, and various other diseases that are linked to poor diet, there is still much debate on whether or not food addiction exists. Some experts in the field of nutrition classify food addictions, emotional eating, and binge eating as all separate disorders, but I believe they are all manifestations of the same problem—with each disorder lying on a different part of the same spectrum. For this reason, I use the terms *food addiction, emotional eating*, and *binge eating* interchangeably.

In my early career, I was the co-owner of a large, multi-disciplinary wellness clinic in Vancouver, British Columbia. It was in this environment and at this point in my life when I really began to appreciate that true healing, of any kind, requires a holistic approach. It became so apparent that, in order to solve the puzzle of my food addiction, I needed to not only study the physical, emotional, and spiritual aspects of addiction, but to truly understand and appreciate the deeply complex relationship between and among food, the mind, the body, and the metaphysical self.

I began to understand that I needed to learn how to re-establish the innate connection between ourselves and Mother Nature; that relationship, one we are all born with but have been trained from infancy to reject, has been around for hundreds of thousands of years. It is this connection between our mind, body, and nature that allowed us to have an intrinsic sense of which foods were good for us and which foods would do us harm. It is only within the past century that we have equated birthdays to cake, Christmas to pie, Easter to chocolate, and after-dinner to dessert. It is for this very reason that I do not write meal plans for my clients, as I believe there is nothing more disempowering to an individual who is on his/her own unique wellness journey. Instead, it is my desire to assist my clients with eliminating toxicities or deficiencies in their thoughts, lifestyle, or diet that are hindering them from maintaining a strong connection with nature, thus enabling them to become their own healers. In addition, I have studied human behaviour under some of the world's greatest masterminds, with a keen interest in grasping why it is that we do all the seemingly unexplainable things we do.

I have written this book from the perspective of an individual who has had firsthand experience with the daunting obstacle of destructive relationship with food and has been able to effectively overcome it. I also have the perspective of a holistic health professional who has committed her career to enabling and encouraging others to achieve that very same goal, by developing a revolutionary, science-based program that streamlines that goal in only 90 days. I believe that each person will take a unique lesson and experience from this book, and because I have not yet had a chance to meet with you, I cannot guarantee what that will be for you.

What I do know is this: If 30 years ago, someone fed me the information I am about to present to you, I would have been spared a tremendous amount of heartache and pain. It's for this reason that I have chosen to share it with the world now. I hope you enjoy reading it as much as I have enjoyed writing it.

Be sure to consult with a medical professional throughout your journey. There are a variety of cognitive behaviour techniques that can be very effective. If you believe you suffer from any mental health condition, speak with your medical doctor about your concerns. If you are currently on any medication, do not discontinue use without your doctor's prior approval.

CHAPTER 1

Recognition

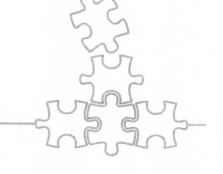

It is no revelation that the true first step to overcoming any addiction is identifying that you are indeed addicted. In saying that, this book is not about steps. Nor is this chapter about that critical first step. In all legitimacy, whether you like it or not, the very fact that you are reading the words on this page is a great indicator that at least a part of you has already surrendered to the notion that you have an unhealthy relationship with food and that you are, in fact, an emotional eater. But, for the sake of being thorough, let's just start by verifying what you may already know.

<u>12 Questions to assess if you have an unhealthy relationship with food</u>

- Do you obsess over or constantly think about your next meal or snack?
- Do you, on a daily basis, eat at least one thing that makes you feel guilty?
- Do you use food as either a reward or punishment?
- Do you often eat when you are not hungry?

- Is food your greatest source of pleasure and pain in your life?
- Do you eat in private, or hide what you are eating from the public because you feel shame?
- Have you ever stolen food from somebody else?
- Do you often regret your food choices, but still repeat them again?
- Do you have a daily ritual that provokes eating when you're not hungry?
- Do you keep a constant supply of your favourite treats in your house, car, or office?
- Do you use food to escape moods and feelings?
- Are your food choices leading to poorer health, but you feel powerless to change them?

If you answered yes to three or more of these, then you have developed an unhealthy eating habit that will continue until you make the definite decision to change it.

For some of you, this may come as no surprise, and many others may only be realizing the magnitude of the problem for the first time. Regardless of which of the two categories you fall under, it is never easy for any of us to face the notion that somewhere down the line, we have lost control. I could not be more sympathetic to your position if this is you, but I also know that it's not my sympathy you need right now. Rather, my guidance will be of much greater service to you at this stage of your life.

Now that we have clearly established some telltale signs of a food addiction, let's move forward and acknowledge that food addictions are incredibly tricky. Why? Because not only is food a socially acceptable coping mechanism, it has been granted the opportunity to seduce us at every checkout aisle, television commercial, bus stop, social gathering, and pretty much everywhere else we go in our waking life. Couple that with the fact that the root of this destructive weed has multiple origins, and they all must be brought to light simultaneously.

To recognize the face of your addiction is to view all its dimensions at once. You can fall victim to the statement, "I have tried everything and nothing works," if you have examined each of its features only one at a time while turning a blind eye to the other facets of this enslavement.

Part 1

Becoming familiar with your personal addiction to food by identifying the triggers and examining the cravings is the difference between fighting a battle with your eyes closed and, well... not.

When you think about it, there is no particular task too hard to address if we break it down and address it in small parts first. Looking at the entire entity as a whole can seem quite daunting to anybody. So, to give ourselves a confident advantage from the beginning, we are going to start by dissecting this piece by piece.

Here, I invite you to take an inventory of your life and simply note all of the common environmental influences—actions, time of day, or places that your cravings routinely surface—and then write them all down on a piece of blank paper or in a workbook. Just write every one that comes to mind in a list. Any order will do.

Anytime you are not actually hungry, but realize you have an impulsive urge to reach for food, note the commonalities between each of the impulses. Mark down where you are, who is around you, what time of day it is, what you have just seen or smelt, what you have just experienced or are about to experience, the activity you are doing, or any other environmental factor that makes it more likely for you to pick up comfort foods.

Become familiar with every detail of the addiction so when the time comes, you can address each craving specifically. There are different reasons behind each and every one of these itches, and I am telling you with confidence that unveiling the answers is entirely within your reach. Over the course of the book, you will gain insight into each of these reasons, then you will be able to discern what you personally need to draw from these insights to overcome your personal eating enigma.

For a series of behaviours to ultimately form a habit, three things are required: 1) a cue (or a trigger); 2) a routine (pattern or practice); and 3) a reward (or payoff). The trigger can be almost anything, ranging from a visual cue, a place, an emotion, a group of individuals, a specific scent, a certain taste, and pretty much everything else in between. Habits are the brain's ingenious way of conserving effort. Instead of having to relearn routines each time we carry them out, our most common tasks become subconscious programs.

Any cue followed by a routine that leads to some kind of payoff can be subconsciously memorized — whether the reward continues to be of service to the individual or not. This prompt doesn't necessarily have to be related to the payoff at all; the cue can also become associated with the reward through mere repetition. For example, a train stop has nothing to do with soft drinks, but if you happened to go to the same train stop each day, and saw an advertisement for your favourite beverage, then went to purchase one from the nearest vending machine and then drank it on several occasions, and then one day the advertisement was removed, merely approaching the station itself could be the new cue that sets the body in motion to seek the reward—the beverage. Ultimately, it comes down to this—the greater the payoff, the more eager the brain is to store it as a habit.

Addiction, however, has nothing to do with enjoyment anymore. Once one is addicted to a specific reward, the behaviours that play out to obtain the payoff and the substance itself can both prove to be devastating to the individual's welfare. In one set of experiments, researchers conditioned mice to respond to certain cues by pressing on a lever and then the mice were rewarded with food. Once this habit was developed, the researchers then poisoned the food, causing the mice to become violently ill; or the mice were electrocuted by the floor of the cage as they walked towards the reward. Once the mice knew the food and floor were dangerous, they stayed away. But when the mice saw the old cues, they automatically pressed the lever and ate the food, or walked across the cage, even though they got sick from the poisonous food or were shocked by the floor. This experiment demonstrates how powerful habits can be once they have been ingrained. It is the environmental trigger that generates the craving and subsequently sets off the compulsive behaviours. Therefore, to create real and long-lasting change, it is imperative to recognize every single one of your personal triggers.

While doing this exercise, I observed myself over the course of a few days and identified that one of my many triggers was simply walking through the door of my home. As a child, as soon as we arrived home from school, my sister and I were each allowed two cookies and a glass of milk. We would religiously grab two place mats from the cabinet, lay them down on the living room floor, and eat our cookies with pure delight while we watched our favourite after-school shows. We looked forward to this moment each day, as it was a time for bonding with each other while we discussed our day. It's a memory I am quite fond of actually.

We had performed this ritual so often that the habit to eat something when I got home became an impulse for me, and over the course of my life, the impulse organically ripened into a full-blown compulsion. Eventually, the act became so ingrained, the desire would fire off on its own accord without any conscious thought, and quite often before I'd even reached my front door. In fact, once I really started to tune into my triggers, I recognized that in my car on the way home there was often a little prelude, where a much more subtle impulse would set the stage; I would find myself in the car carelessly daydreaming about what I intended to pull from the cupboard upon arriving home. This was once a conscious action that eventually reformed into an unconscious program, one that I had let run on autopilot for over 20 years. It had been granted so much airtime that I no longer even noticed it, much less recognized that it ran the show.

In Chapter 4, we will become better acquainted with the neurological programming that allows a harmless little habit to refine itself into an unassuming impulse and then ultimately grow into a beastly compulsion, but for now, the focus is simply recognition. Take the time now to become intimate with your food addiction by identifying all the external environmental factors that trigger each and every craving. Allow yourself to take an account of your personal triggers—including all of the foods that trigger you to binge uncontrollably—so that eventually you can work at being one step ahead of the addiction, just like any true master needs to be. This activity may take some time and you will find yourself coming back to add to the list as the days go by. There's no set number for how many cues you'll need to identify, or even a limit to reach; the goal is simply to recognize each of them and note the commonalities between them.

Part 2

There's something else that you need to become very familiar with, and that is yourself. As cliché as that sounds, there's absolutely no way around it when it comes to your healing. I am not simply referring to that familiarity you feel when you catch your reflection as you pass a window. That picture you see in the mirror is merely a collective image of mostly the dead parts of you. Behind that mask is who you really are, and beneath the soil is where you truly reside. Beyond the borders of your skin, nails, and hair, there is an entire universe filled with a wonder of biochemical reactions, electrical impulses, and even countless life forms that too often we are completely unenlightened to.

We tend to get so caught up with the outside world that it limits us from ever taking an account of the world within us. When we neglect our personal universe by turning our senses solely outward to the external environment, it makes it appear more real than the inner world. We, in turn, become deaf to subtle cries within the body. It is not uncommon for the body to try and get our attention with a mighty roar, an emotion so violent it can't be ignored. The feeling can consume you with such vigour that the instinct will naturally be to desperately reach for something outside of you to calm the storm within you.

Just like our external environmental triggers, we need to recognize our internal emotional triggers as well. Unfortunately, this task is usually met with much greater resistance. That is because, to a great majority of us, suppressing emotions is a much more common practice. I might even go so far as to say that numbing oneself is often one of the primary goals when emotional eating, whereas giving ourselves the permission to feel the full spectrum of emotions has become a much more foreign act—one heavily frowned upon in today's society, at a huge detriment to our physical and emotional health.

In terms of our wellbeing, drawing our senses inward is a necessary practice with abundant rewards that are always available to all of us, when and if we choose. Like any other practice, the art is refined over time, and we inevitably get better at it with enough rehearsal. With regular repetition, it too can grow into a habit, and eventually birth a whole new way of being. Removing judgment and recognizing the emotion just before every impulse is crucial and our focus at this stage, but becoming intimate with your internal universe as a whole is where the real power lies. By the end of the book, you'll understand and appreciate exactly why.

Just as you listed triggers earlier in this chapter, I now encourage you to list the corresponding emotional cues that lead you to compulsively eat. Record each thought that you attempt to silence with food, and make the distinction between hunger and nourishment versus misery and self-soothing. Stick with it! I know at times it may seem grim and appear pointless, but that perception couldn't be further from the truth.

Recognizing yourself doesn't stop there. It's pointless to know what plagues and disheartens you if you don't also recognize what fuels and inspires you to an equal degree. It's not unjust to claim that being oblivious to your true values makes you even more vulnerable to addiction due to the powerful neurotransmitter dopamine.

Dopamine has a bit of a bad reputation when it comes to addiction, but dopamine itself is not the enemy. Often when we hear someone referring to a person with a substance abuse problem, they would call that person a "dope addict," as if that were a bad thing. What many of us don't realize is, we are all "dope addicts" to some degree. If it were not for this incredibly motivating little chemical, none of us would ever do anything.

Dopamine is a neurochemical associated with reward, and is crucial for motivating and directing goal-seeking behaviour. Dopamine also regulates thought, movement, attention, mood, and learning. Low levels of the chemical will cause you to be easily distracted, unfocused, and even feel depressed, which is why it's associated with attention deficit disorder (ADD).

Things are only perceived as important or valuable to you if they activate your dopamine neurons. Once dopamine is released, it then provokes action, and also continues to reinforce the same behaviour. For example, the sight and smell of a chocolate cake may be the cues that activate dopamine neurons, generating a craving for the cake, which will lead you to eat it. The taste of the cake releases even more dopamine, ensuring you continue to eat the entire slice, or maybe even help yourself to seconds.

The cake itself would not create a craving if the brain didn't have prior experience with this specific, delicious reward. Cravings form once a cue is associated with a payoff, and cravings do not subside until the payoff has been obtained. The payoff may come in the form of a cake, but it could represent a variety of potential rewards. This reward, which is camouflaged as dessert, could be rooted from a desire to remedy boredom, a need for increased energy, or a longing to be comforted, among many other things.

We are visual animals. So an advertisement for, let's say, pizza, can release enough dopamine to shift your entire focus towards retrieving that pizza. Pizza could have been the last thing on your mind before you saw the advert, but all of a sudden it's as if your thoughts become possessed by the idea of eating it. This process is the rationale for visualising your goals, writing them down, and then marking them off once they have been achieved. Dopamine is released just by ticking off one of your attained goals on a list. The more dopamine a particular goal releases, the more valuable the brain perceives that goal to be, and the more likely it is to become a habit (or a subconscious practice).

Everything we do is related to this powerful chemical. It used to be that the activities that gave us the greatest pleasure were the ones we needed to do in order to survive and to further reproduce — the pursuit of food and the desire for sex are at the pinnacle of that list. If we were eating the meal plan that was provided to us by Mother Earth, then we would be unlikely to develop an unhealthy obsession with food because — although the desire for any food can have an effect on dopamine — it is the engineered foods created by the food industry that release a surplus of dopamine. These artificially designed foods deliver much greater rewards (dopamine) than the foods naturally occurring in nature.

The potency of a stimulant is what can create an addiction. It's believed that our brains can safely handle between 100 to 300 units of dopamine at one time.[1] If a food or stimulant releases excessive doses of dopamine, our dopamine receptors in the brain down-regulate to compensate, making us less sensitive to dopamine, and in turn, we need more of the stimulant to get a similar pleasurable feeling. Junk foods, engineered by the food industry, are catering to this problem much the same way the porn industry is attributed to an unhealthy and destructive appetite for sex.

Food, drugs, sex, gambling, and shopping all have the ability to release large amounts of dopamine, but so does everything else we truly desire. It's going after or obtaining the things in life that we desire the most that gives us a great surge of dopamine. As a result, we feel motivated to keep going.

In regards to emotional eating, foods like fat and sugar happen to be among the things we desire the most, but simply because we allowed ourselves to chase that goal more than any other goal in our lifetime. Our clever brain has memorized food to be the quickest and easiest route to get its dope fix.

If we aren't spending our time pursuing inspiring goals and going after the things in life that we innately desire, we deprive ourselves of the release of dopamine, which consequently increases our need to get it from an alternate substance, such as food. Before modern-day agriculture, we had to hunt and gather our food. In those times, we would have to go searching for food, which was not an immediate guarantee. This is in great contrast to the luxuries of our present day. It makes sense that the prospect of finding food releases large amounts of dopamine because if we waited till we felt hunger, it might be too late.

With such vast amounts of food readily available to us, we have transcended some of the dilemmas our ancestors faced. However, now we have created an entirely new problem, in that we must replace hunting for food and getting our dopamine fix with other profitable daily quests. Without a goal that matters to you as an individual, you will be subject to the constant pursuit of food.

When we have a goal that is sincerely valuable to us, and then we see the prospect of that goal and/or we achieve it, dopamine will be released, allowing us to feel motivated and excited to keep striving for it. The reward is the burst of dopamine along with the good feelings it evokes within you.

The opposite is also true; if you are filling your life with actions that are meaningless to you, or perhaps you lack direction and goals in your life—ones that are honestly inspiring to you—the result will naturally be lower levels of dopamine being released in the brain. As a by-product of living an unstimulating life, you are at risk of feeling depressed and unmotivated to do anything, except, of course, eat food for the sake of that dopamine fix. Being ignorant to our desires and unaware of our personal values can cause us to feel directionless, which in turn makes us more susceptible to reaching for an addictive substance to lift us from our depressed state.

In the case of emotional eating, our subconscious has been programmed from repetition and past experience that food will always give us that necessary dopamine fix. In other words, we need dopamine, and without a goal to attain that comes from a place of inspiration, the instinct will always be to get our hit from wherever the brain has learned from past experience that it can get it from. The holy grail in your healing will be determining what else in your life lights a fire and instigates you to take actions other than the usual trip to the fridge.

If you have truly been digesting all of this information, then you may protest at this stage and say to me that if you had any idea at all what ignited a spark and kindled the flame within you, then you wouldn't be looking for your dopamine fix in your pantry; you wouldn't be addicted to food in the first place, and you would most likely tell me that you wouldn't have picked up this book. To be fair, a statement like that does have some validity. But don't mistake what I am saying here; I'm not blind to the reality that many feel desperately lost in a world that appears to have little to no meaning. It is the effects of that hopelessness that I have become so intimate with, the understanding that the absence of a real purpose is a direct link to so much of our human suffering, and the common denominator in many of our lives.

I have absolutely no expectation that just because I have shared this information with you, you will magically have a revelation in this moment to what is truly important to you and your life. It would be erroneous to expect that of anybody. I do, however, encourage you to have the expectation that by the end of our time together—should you allow yourself to finish, to be open to change and do the work—then you will have confidence in your own life's mission (subject to being refined over time, of course). You will be well-versed on your highest values in your current life, and you will recognize the source of the light within you.

CHAPTER 2

Appreciation

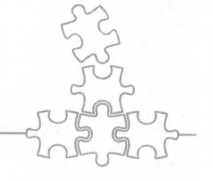

Appreciation is key, but I'm not just talking about appreciating the mind, the body, or what's on our plates. Without question, those are important aspects and well-known concepts, for a valid reason. Yet, as truthful as it is that you must learn to appreciate yourself and your life to overcome emotional eating patterns, not everyone knows the direct route to Love-Yourselfville. If we all had a clear map of where and how to lay down the track to arrive at that destination, then compulsive eating wouldn't be such a prevailing issue, now would it? Let's be genuine here. If you are not currently in a state of love and gratitude for yourself and your life, then there must be some kind of blockage, even if you have not yet identified what that block is.

In fairness to you and to every attempt you have ever made, it's not as though you can simply get up one morning, look yourself dead in the mirror, and tell yourself that you love your body, your life, your thoughts, your environment, and expect to suddenly and honestly feel that way. It would be beyond unrealistic to expect that of yourself, and of your life as a whole. As much as we are addicted to the idea of selling each other this fantasy, it simply doesn't work that way. If old beliefs or emotions still remain, then you will inevitably fall back to familiar thoughts and habits, and you will continue to feel resentment for yourself, your body, your actions, your plate, and perhaps even your emotional state. You won't believe the words you are saying in the mirror anyhow, and the entire act becomes inconsequential.

In all honesty, it is also not unreasonable for you to feel worse after your brief pep talk, as you stare straight in that mirror knowing that you just flat-out lied to yourself. You might even start to give yourself grief for not feeling how you believe you are "supposed" to feel in life. Maybe there's a moment of shame as you recognize that yet one more desperate attempt at positive thinking has turned out to be nothing more than another loss in your seemingly endless list of efforts and defeats to break free from your misery. You have just risked allowing a deep sense of failure to cast a shadow upon your entire day, and, as you acknowledge that you don't miraculously feel any different on the inside, you are now left standing face-to-face with the fear that you might not ever really change your state of being.

After spending all that time in front of the mirror praising and criticizing yourself, you're not only late for work, your outfit kind of makes you look fat, you're starving, and there's not enough time to change your clothes and also prepare something healthy to eat. At this stage, a cascade of emotions runs through you, including a sense of total disempowerment. Perhaps out of a desire to feel a moment of relief from that recent and epic failure, you allow the thought, *Maybe I should just have one of those two chocolate chip muffins sitting in the fridge,* to pass through your mind. *At least that muffin has the power to make me feel good, even if only temporarily*. There are not a lot of conscious thoughts or actions that take place between that initial thought and the moment when you are having thoughts of regret while you stare at a paper lining that was once wrapped around a chocolate chip muffin.

Now you're really in trouble, as it tasted pretty damn good, and evidently, you have no control anyhow. Clearly, your attempts are futile, and there is no sense in holding back now, not while you're still pretty hungry and you have one more really delicious muffin that's ready to eat in the fridge. If this sounds familiar to you, then you might also know from repeated experience that the food selections for the remainder of the day will likely be sequential to the first—all reflecting a steady stream of consoling oneself while succumbing to delicious temptations. Thoughts like, *I have already failed at my new life today, so I might as well live it up and eat as much as I want; I'll start fresh tomorrow*. Or lies like, "There's no point, I will never break the cycle anyway, and at least this dessert will make me happy," become so loud they are mistaken as truth, and as a result, the vicious cycle is given the authority to continue on.

Despite what you have convinced yourself of for all these years, you are not alone in this battle, and what you're experiencing is not as abnormal as you might have led yourself to believe. There are perfectly logical explanations for all of this, and over the course of this book, I will share them with you. My intention is for you to be able to use these explanations to decipher how, over a long period of time, your brain and body adapted to your current state of being. And, as a bonus, with just as much dedication to this new direction, you can work towards an entirely new way of thinking, feeling, and being.

Granted, if you gazed at yourself in the mirror every morning and said loving words as a ritual, then it could very well have a significant impact long-term, but we don't often make it that far along that path because of roadblocks or aspects we haven't yet examined— which, of course, I will discuss in more detail in the following chapters.

You are only human, and you know little more in life than what you have real experience with. It's not hard to give up on setting new habits when you feel completely powerless to deeply instilled old habits that have been there for pretty much as long as you can remember, and with no real sense that your reality could ever be any different. Why would you believe these affirmations if you have not yet seen any evidence in your life that you truly have authority over these compulsions? We need to experience some kind of evidence that we have the potential to mandate all of our food choices in order to make a long-term change. Without that wisdom, at the first sign of failure or undue hardship, any excuse will do to convince us that our efforts are a waste of time.

It is time to take the power back, or perhaps admit you never really lost any of your power in the first place. Yes, that's right, there's a twist.

This chapter on appreciation is focused on gaining perspective from a whole new corner of the room. I am suggesting we learn to appreciate the habit itself! If this is where I lost you, then allow me a moment to explain. I recognize that initially, this approach may seem coun- terintuitive, but I assure you it's not, by any means. I understand that this idea may seem foreign, and with it could come the false illusion that if you learn to appreciate it, then you might not ever stop it—let me comfort you by telling you that's not the case.

You absolutely have the ability to decide that you no longer have a use for something in your life and admit it's time to let it go while acknowledging why you ever invited it into your world in the first place. It's also okay to admit the benefits of your life that led you to repeatedly call upon it, so much so that it became a routine. Understanding why it consequently became a habit and distinguishing what was gained by you repeatedly giving it the opportunity to manifest into an authoritative compulsion within the body enables you to finally and truly take control.

Let's stop to think about it. The primary objective here is to take over a force that has gotten very much out of control. Anything in your life that you resent—or are infatuated with, for that matter—you also give the power to run you. Grant yourself permission to acknowledge that at each stage of your food addiction, you made these decisions because that was what you needed in that time and space. Honour those choices, because by doing so, you are also honouring yourself. One can never truly empower themselves to make new, definite decisions unless they freely admit that they chose to give in to emotional eating merely because it benefitted them each and every time to do so.

Through this exercise, you will regain trust in your decisions and develop the understanding that you can and will be able to give new choices just as much power, if you see how they can serve you to an equal or greater degree. Concede in this moment that perhaps you are the great designer of your own life; see how you have been making perfect decisions all this time. The aim here is to shift your perspective onto the enigma and view it from a higher understanding. It is now time to confess to yourself that you have actually been completely in charge, albeit at some stage you fell asleep. Once you allow yourself to do this, you become armed with just enough confidence that you can now imagine yourself reaching for the reigns of your wild and unstable horse. Without that necessary self-assurance, you wouldn't be in a state where you believe wholeheartedly that you have the supremacy to demand a change of direction.

Please don't try and take a shortcut and cheat yourself here. It's really not enough to look back at your life and perceive only a few perks to your world in terms of your emotional eating, and then move on without really allowing yourself to grasp this concept. Sure, listing only some of the profits gives you the gist, but only getting the essence of something is much less meaningful than having a full experience.

Let's say you were about to have surgery, and you could choose from two different surgeons to perform the operation. Doctor #1 has learned how to do the surgery. She gets the idea logically, but has no real past experience performing it. Doctor #2 knows the procedure and has also performed the surgery before. Which of these two are you more likely to choose? If you have selected the second surgeon—and I really hope you have—it is because you understand that there is a significant variance between simply knowing philosophy versus experiencing it.

To understand a concept without experience means you have solely learned the philosophy while robbing yourself of the emotions we feel during the experience.

Emotionally valuable information is easier to remember, so a deeply emotional experience is required to make a lasting change. To learn a philosophy while permitting yourself to also have an experience increases the likelihood of both a positive physiological change and the prospect of long-term impact.

You have made the decision every single time you reached for food; you did so because it served you in some capacity, otherwise, you would not have done it. Merely understanding this as though it might be true is not akin to feeling the emotional shift when you know that without a doubt, it is guaranteed to be true. Additionally, simply getting the gist of this idea means you'll miss yet another, and no less impressive, result of the exercise that we cover in Chapter 3. Unfortunately, there is no shortcut in your healing. The only way out starts with true and meaningful revelations in your thinking and feelings.

At first, this may take some creative thinking; it's not easy to admit that you've gained something from that which you have resented for so long. But the less you resent it, the higher the likelihood that you can see its true nature, and the more you can see the legitimacy of the choice to have it in your life for so long. So, begin by listing the additional payoffs (besides the seductive tastes), and allow yourself to wake up to the reality that you're still very much in the driver's seat.

One by one, go down a list and write as many benefits as you can think of as to how your eating behaviours and the food itself benefitted all of the aspects of your life. Initially, you—like most everyone else—might struggle with this exercise because of your deep-seated resentment towards your compulsive eating, and that is completely understandable. Your mind will repeatedly try and go back to ruminating over all the different ways your erratic eating patterns have ruined your life. Yes, of course, there are drawbacks; if there weren't, you would not be seeking to be released from its grip. For the sake of your healing, please try and focus on the goal, which is to appreciate the habit for everything it has done *for* you as well. You need to silence that voice of resentment—you hear enough of it day to day—and focus on gratitude for each experience instead.

When you forbid yourself from having any other feeling beyond resentment for something that is in your life, consequently, you are putting yourself at risk to reaching for whatever has the ability to numb these feelings—in this case, food. In all honesty, it's not the food that is to blame. We all eat food, but not everyone has a grudge against it. It's the abusive relationship with food that is actually the source of the stress. Resenting the food has, to date, done nothing more than give you something to harbor bad feelings over. This quote from Albert Einstein (BrainyQuote.com) is fitting: "We cannot solve our problems by using the same level of thinking we used when we created them." It's time to give up the cynicism so you can trade it in for empowerment.

I now encourage you to recall as many memories about food as you possibly can—the more the better. Allow yourself to relive the moment, and then write down as many benefits as you can possibly come up with. Get creative, and ask yourself the questions you need to in order to understand why it has become such a significant crutch in your life.

- How did your past and present food choices influence your world spiritually?
- What has been the advantage to you mentally?
- Did convenient snack foods allow more time for study during university?
- Does food remedy boredom?
- Did high-sugar treats give you a kick during times of study?
- Did not paying attention to your nutrition needs allow for more time focusing on other things?
- How have unhealthy food choices propelled you in your line of work?
- Do you work in a fast-paced environment that made it more convenient to just eat whatever was quick and available?
- Are regular dinner meetings with clients a part of your everyday routine?
- Does eating chocolate console you during stressful situations?
- Does sharing a piece of cake at the end of the day allow you to bond with your partner?
- Is it easier for you to eat whatever your family eats?
- Does your partner also have uncontrolled eating, and that's something you do together?
- Does going out for dessert give you something to do with your friends?
- Does it take your mind off things when you feel overwhelmed?
- Does it keep you preoccupied when you feel lonely?

I could keep going, but I am sure you get the point. There are thousands of possibilities that I could list, but each of them is unique to our own lives. If you need to, you can refer to Chapter 1 and revert back to a moment when you experienced each of those triggers. Go to each memory and look for viable justification for why you gave in at each of these times. Without the complete understanding of why you are doing it, you will never be able to identify what else you can do besides more eating to give you an equal or greater benefit.

Once a habit is formed, it can't be eradicated; it can only be updated. It wouldn't be very useful if you forgot how to ride a bike every time you stopped riding it for a few days, or even a few years. So, once our foot hits the pedal again, the body can perform the memorized routine that gets you from point A to point B.

Now, if you were in the habit of riding your bike to work every morning, leaving your home could cue you to subconsciously walk over to your bike, jump on it, and you'd eventually find yourself at work without much conscious effort. Let's say that you decided you'd like to get in the habit of driving your new car to work instead. You could replace the habit of leaving your home and riding the bike to work with leaving your home and driving a car to get there. The cue and the desired payoff may always stay the same, but the practice can be refined or replaced. You can appreciate now why it is so essential to acknowledge what the specific payoffs are that you are truly trying to attain.

CHAPTER 3

Surrogacy

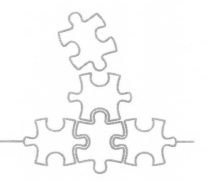

Y ou could try to refrain from old eating habits by using willpower alone, but you will inevitably fall prey to its limitations. Willpower is an incredibly deceptive little bugger. It appears to work so effectively a good portion of the time, but then it seems to fail miserably when we need it the most. Have you ever wondered why it is that at times it's so remarkably reliable, and then within mere hours so deeply unfaithful?

One of the most confusing things to me along my journey was figuring out why I was unshakable one minute, and mere moments later I'd completely and utterly lose all self-control. It was as though I was two separate people; one person who had no issue with saying no—and with incredible conviction, at that—and then a whole other person who basically had the ability to resist temptation to the degree of a two-year-old child. Searching for some logic behind my erratic behavior became a mission, so I went digging through textbooks high and low.

All that digging eventually led me to learn how willpower works in the brain, and just what kind of limits it actually has. Willpower works similarly to a muscle—the more you use it, the stronger it gets. But just like a muscle, it can become drained and fatigued with overuse. Exercising willpower actually depletes a lot of mental energy. Without that spare energy, it no longer has the fuel it needs to continue doing its job.

It works similarly to the battery on your phone. It has a point at which it must be recharged, and the more you use the phone, the sooner you will need to recharge. So it stops what it's doing and becomes inactive, until of course, it's been restored. Willpower really doesn't care where you are or what you think you have committed to overcoming; when it's done, it's done, and you won't be able to count on it for quite some time.

In order to restore willpower, you need two things— food and rest. So basically, when you're tired, hungry, and it's time to make a decision about what to eat, that is the moment when you need its defences the most. But it's also highly likely going to be in conjunction with when it'll abandon you to battle alone.

In 1998, a study was published wherein psychologist Roy Baumeister demonstrated an experiment. He brought subjects into a room in front of an oven with chocolate cookies inside it. The delicious scent of cookies filled up the room. A bowl of radishes was also placed in the room, and then half of the subjects were told they could eat as many radishes as they wanted, but the cookies were off limits. The remaining half of the subjects were permitted to consume as many cookies as they desired. Afterward, both groups were given 30 minutes to solve a tricky geometric puzzle. Baumeister and his colleagues found that people who ate radishes (and resisted the cookies) gave up on the puzzle almost twice as fast as those who did not have to resist the cookies. It appeared from this clever experiment that drawing on willpower to resist the cookies weakened the subjects' self-control for subsequent situations and further problem-solving.

The act of repeated decision-making can also affect how much energy our brain expends; in stressful situations, creative initiatives, interacting with others, resisting urges to speak up, or even forcing yourself to smile around your mother-in-law, are all tasks that are energy-expending as well. These operations take from the same supply as willpower, leading to even lower fuel stores at a much faster rate.

Various factors have a significant impact on how quickly one experiences willpower fatigue. Spending a great deal of time and energy on daily tasks that are uninspiring to you not only pose a threat in terms of dopamine levels, but they can also contribute to the rate at which you experience willpower fatigue.

In one experiment on willpower depletion, Kathleen Vohs, PhD, and colleagues, of the University of Minnesota, found that those who were told to persuade a hostile audience that they were "likable" endured willpower fatigue substantially more so than those who were allowed to act naturally toward to audience.

What's really valuable to note here is that willpower can't always be counted on, especially in the instance of resisting certain foods. Recharging our battery with sleep alone is simply not enough. Research shows that glucose stores play a large part in this game. Evidence suggests that a huge factor in whether or not one suffers from willpower depletion might be due to low levels of glucose, and might have less to do with lack of sleep or physical exhaustion. Prior to asking her study subjects to suppress their emotional reactions to a video clip, Kathleen Vohs took half of her subjects and had them endure 24 hours of sleep deprivation. They were then tested on their strength of self-control. Oddly, she found that those who'd been sleep deprived were no more at risk of willpower depletion than those who'd had a good night's rest.

This insight is integral to making any kind of long-term change. If self-control is not at our disposal, it needs time and fuel to be replenished, and that means we need an additional *something* in lieu of its absence. We have to accept that in order to go the long haul in our healing and to have any real success, we must be able to count on something more sustainable than willpower alone.

Willpower is often used as the primary defence in the face of temptations, making this one of the reasons addictions appear to be so laborious to overcome. It makes sense then that the more you desire something, someone, or a particular food, the more often and the more fiercely you will use willpower to avoid succumbing to it, and the quicker you will use up willpower stores. It then becomes inevitable that you will eventually exhaust your willpower and be left standing completely defenceless in the face of your seductress.

Sugar was my seductress, and I can say with certainty that I know I am definitely not alone. If you are one of the countless people who understands the importance of clean eating, but the ability to avoid junk food eludes you, and you can't actually make good decisions for any significant period of time when it comes to your meal plan, then you are highly likely a victim of repeated willpower fatigue. If you, like so many others, have ever broken a promise to yourself about adopting a healthier lifestyle—or if you have a habit of binging on something you've repeatedly vowed to quit—then you now know the culprit.

Binging on food is an impending fate when we suppress our food desire for a period of time, or if we deprive ourselves of adequate nutrition and/or rest. Learning this was pivotal in my wellness journey because, for me, in order to govern my desires, I needed to become familiar with them.

So then, how does one escape from this destructive maze of the mind?

The key is planted within each and every one of us.

There is no way outside of your mind and body—they are your forever home. If you feel trapped inside it, that's because the real you that lives in your little secret garden has been buried deep down within a jungle of weeds.

I've found that the only way forward is to harvest a greater desire that not only trumps the old one (in this case, the desire to eat comforting foods), but the height of the new desire must tower over the old one significantly. The new goal must be so substantial to you as an individual that it beats the old desire by an absolute landslide. It is essential that it conflicts considerably with the old desires—the one you have become an unarmed prisoner to. You need to ambush the food addiction by eradicating your deep longing for unhealthy food and replace that longing for something deeper that is waiting patiently for you to allow it to grow inside you.

If you are using willpower to avoid something, then that's a great indicator that you still have a longing for it, and perhaps you haven't yet linked a greater goal to put down the old one for. Simply put, you have not yet allowed yourself the gift of admitting you have a more valuable, enjoyable, or meaningful reward to live for, strive for, and be as healthy as possible for.

It's no secret that proper nutrition is a biological need. We have just learned how denying oneself of that need means we're likely doomed for binging. On the same note, a reason to live and the satiating rewards of achieving your life's goals is an aspect that also needs to be fulfilled. Your mind and body can detect a void in that area, and that void will give way to finding fulfillment by any other means it can.

Without having something else that excites you besides food, you're playing a losing game. Imagine that you're experiencing willpower fatigue, then you see or smell freshly baked cookies. If you have no other thing to turn to in that moment that's just as sweet for you (I'm not referring solely to taste), something that provokes just as much or even more dopamine to be released, then it'll be mere moments before you have a face full of chocolate chip cookies.

In my opinion, the purpose of life is to love and create. Whether what one creates is in the form of a child, a business, art, a book, a garden, a service, or anything else we desire to put out in the universe—we all have an intrinsic drive to create. We need something to propel us forward. We (in the Western world) are fortunate enough to be fairly free to choose whatever we feel truly inspired to create. As one part physical being, it's to your advantage to conceive that your body is a vessel—one that is perfectly designed to create something extraordinary in this world. You can use your time, expend your energy, and take up space to create whatever you please, but only to the limit of what you believe to be a possibility for you. If you do not trust in yourself or your gifts, you will feel too handicapped by these doubts to produce anything of any more significance to you than an external dependency.

By now, you can better understand why your new goal can't just be any old goal; it needs to be an inner burning desire from within you that holds more weight than any other desire you've ever dreamt of having in the past. The idea of obtaining this goal needs to lift your spirits like nothing before. Not your mother's spirit, your partner's, your neighbour's, your best friend's, or even the pastor's at the local church.

Mark Muraven, PhD, and colleagues, of the University at Albany, found that subjects who felt compelled to exert self-control for the sake of what others wanted were more easily depleted than people who allowed their own goals and desires to be a driving force. Baumeister, Muraven, and their colleagues also researched the impact of mood on willpower. When subjects were exposed to comedy or gifts, they became more cheerful and they exhibited less willpower fatigue than what was usually displayed after exercising self-control. These and other studies suggest that willpower fatigues faster in the absence of an alternate means of reward.

Just to make it clear, I'm not suggesting that we should all do what we feel like at all hours of the day, without any regard for the consequences to our loved ones and the rest of society. I am merely pointing out that suppressing who you really are, injecting other people's beliefs about your life into your mind, and living by what others think you should be doing means you are living with no regard to the consequences for yourself—which does an equal disservice to our world. If you have a greater goal that's important to you and that goal rewards you in some way while simultaneously serving humanity, as far as I am concerned, you're doing just as well as anybody.

It's almost a cruel joke that the element that often dictates what we desire is what we perceived to be denied in the past. It's safe to assume that you have attempted to deny yourself pleasure from food on repeated occasions; would I be just in saying that? The act of wanting something and denying yourself of it only makes the addiction more robust. An element that can't be avoided is that the desire for the comfort foods, or the lusting after them, needs to be annihilated. I believe the only way to do that is to perceive how your emotional eating and abusive relationship with food is going to get in the way of obtaining your new, much more sacred goal that actually means something to you.

Think of it like becoming a mother. Before the child is conceived, the woman has many things in her life that she gets joy from; but once she finds out she's with child, those things become much less important and her focus is turned towards the baby she's carrying. Her attention becomes focused, and her time and energy for things other than what her baby needs begin to diminish greatly. If she perceives any of those old things that she once loved to be a threat to her new child, she won't think twice about dumping it like an old mattress on the side of the road. What I'm asking of you here is to leave your obsession with junk food in the alley next to that grubby old mattress, while embracing something more meaningful to you.

It doesn't work if you try injecting a new goal that is actually someone else's desire for you, or someone else's desire or habit you have inflicted upon yourself. Demolish the belief that there is a goal you should be going after. Doing a task because you believe you should do it—based on the opinions of those around you—only increases the likelihood of willpower fatigue, because you don't actually want to be doing it. It is important that it be an innate burning desire that inspires you without outside influence.

In order to not abandon the goal you need a constant state, and the energy to power it must come from the infinite source within you. Because of the simple truth that we are the only guaranteed constant thing in our own lives, the new goal must be exclusively fuelled by you. The charge you need to continue to light your flame, to reach for your new life, must come from within or you will impulsively return to old habits every single time, without fail.

In the absence of love and gratitude for your life and who you truly are, and without a real understanding of what's valuable to you, you will never bother to ignite a spark. In this case, procrastinating on goals will be the inevitable fate. You certainly wouldn't be able to see the prospect of a new possibility for yourself if you can't even see how you can trust in yourself to obtain the goal in the first place.

We all have these inner burning desires, but too often we don't believe we deserve them, or we have limiting beliefs holding us back from pursuing them; maybe we feel incapable of obtaining what we really want. Sometimes we can't even admit that we want them out of fear of failure, the belief we aren't smart enough, fear of rejection or judgment of others, or that we aren't destined for greatness. Or maybe that we aren't physically fit or attractive enough. Many factors can lead us to bury these desires, making more room for external addictions. It is for this reason that my program "The Eating Enigma: 90 days to transform your relationship with food" contributes to reprograming individuals on both the conscious and subconscious levels.

I'm not blind to the fact that this is easier said than done, but examining who you are, what you really want in your life, and what you feel you deserve for yourself—and then taking the necessary steps to go after it—may very well be the only way out of the maze. It has been exploring this piece that made me realize how paramount it is to our own personal reality that we each really delve into ourselves. It's what led me to understand how important it really is to "know thyself" while honouring that beautiful individual uniqueness.

In the following chapters, I will expose methods that lead to a greater understanding of your true nature; your innermost desires; your emotions that are cleverly disguised as beliefs about yourself and your life; the fears that cripple you from ever even trying to reach for anything else in life besides food. We will discuss the tools that are available to all of us. These tools will lead you to be able to distinguish the difference between the truth about yourself and your worth, and the lies that have been injected into your mind based on perceptions of past experience. I will systematically share the approach that worked for me and my clients and what it takes to really become familiar with oneself.

In the meantime, my greatest desire for you is to understand why it's so crucial to your healing to be authentic to yourself, and what can be gained by being open to finding your true purpose during your very limited time on earth.

So while you are in this transition phase, armed with the knowledge that you can't count on willpower alone, you'll have to resort to leaning on surrogacy instead, replacing old behaviours and routines with new ones. As time goes by, you can refine this list, allowing this new crutch to not only hold you up, but to uplift you and propel you forward towards your new goals as well.

Remember those triggers you noted in Chapter 1, and the benefits of leaning on food you listed in Chapter 2? Well, what you need now is to come up with other surrogate behaviours and routines for each of those triggers. This will ultimately result in the payoffs you were previously trying to obtain. Make sure to write them down in an easily accessible place, as you may want to refer to them often.

Here are two examples of what I mean.

Example One
Trigger: Driving home from work.
Payoff: Allows me to shift my mental focus away from my work life and stresses of my day.
Surrogates: Listening to an audiobook on health and nutrition. Take a new route home or stop to visit a friend. Think about and plan my weekend.

Example Two
Trigger: Walking through the doors of my home.

Payoff: Helps me unwind.
Surrogates: Walk through the door and head straight for
a bath. Prepare my space to start writing.
Go straight for my yoga mat.

This may seem like a bit of a tedious task, but you will be glad you did it. The next time, you won't have to lean on willpower alone because you will have clearly written out alternatives that can lead you to obtaining similar rewards. Once you have identified what's important in your own life you can refine this list, as I have. Refining this list ensures that those surrogate actions not only abate you from emotional eating, but they go further by bringing you even one step closer to your new, more fulfilling destiny.

When you picked up this book and committed to hearing what I had to say, I know you didn't expect so much homework. Trust me, I have never been a fan of homework myself, but there's no shortcut around this. I repeatedly insist that you write these things down for a wildly impressive reason: When we learn new information, we make new circuits in the brain.

Remembering is sustaining those new connections. So when we learn new information, we gain what we call "semantic memories." Another way we learn information is by having an experience with it. When we include our five senses, our senses send a burst of information from all of their pathways. This gives us a greater chance of remembering that experience in the future. Writing your surrogate actions down works just as your notes did when you were studying for a test in school. It increased the likelihood that you would be able to recall the information while being tested or during a stressful state.

In short, excessive mental exertion and states of low blood sugar (which we will discuss more intimately in Chapter 5) will mean your brain has little or no fuel to expend on willpower. Grasping this concept also provides a clue to why starving oneself is so closely intertwined with bouts of binging.

CHAPTER 4

Admiration

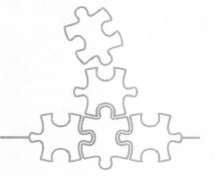

t is vital to understand that no matter what you learn about nutrition, if you don't also learn to love yourself, you will never give the body what it needs. It also makes sense that if we feel an internal void, we will have an incessant compulsion to fill it.

Unfortunately, for a vast majority of us, we have lost sight of where true fulfillment actually comes from. Feeling fulfilled is not about obtaining external goals, people, or things you think you love. It's feeling full on the inside and, from that state, making the decisions that reflect that full feeling. Taking action steps towards the events you believe you deserve. When learning how to master your destiny, you must cultivate change and initiate action from the inside out.

Let me ask you, what is your greatest desire at the present moment?

Now, what is the source of your greatest depression?

Is the source of your greatest depression the fact that you don't have your greatest desire? There's a good chance, if you've read this far, that one of your greatest desires is to be unshackled from the chains of emotional eating.

Take a moment to think about all the justifications you can possibly come up with for why you don't have what you want in life. Every single excuse that comes to mind on why you haven't been able to break free — write them all down.

-
-
-
-
-
-
-
-
-
-

I now want you to think about an accomplishment in your life that you are most proud of — a goal that you have already achieved that you cherish most of all.

Could all of your justifications apply to both cases if you wanted them to?

Whether we achieve a goal is not solely dependent on outside influences—sure, it can have an influence to some degree—but the level to which we take ownership of it has the most authority over a goal's success. Our goals are defenseless against the forces of our beliefs.

It is as simple as that! The excuses are always available to you if you don't believe your situation can truly change. Those reasons have an insignificant influence on the outcome if not fuelled by either faith or fear.

Your current position on the field is the one you are most confident to play. Each of our lives is a direct reflection of what we truly believe we deserve and how prepared we feel to play the game. When I learned how to have unbound admiration for myself and for my life, then I was compelled to admit where I was truly inspired to play on the field. I no longer resented the nature of the game or any person in it.

Obstacles are inevitable on any journey, no matter which path we choose. No one has managed to have any real success in anything in life without enduring some kind of trial to get it. In fact, success or no success, challenges are a part of life for all of us. The real danger when it comes to our goals is our level of deservingness, not the adversity we face pursuing them. The problem arises when we doubt our personal potential to obtain the life we want. When we carry the opinion that we are not deserving of the path we desire, we allow brief times of hardship to stop us dead in our tracks and we settle on an alternative route altogether.

The misconception that we have a limit on what we can create or what we deserve tricks our minds into picking a path that is more familiar to us. We can imagine going down this familiar road because we have seen our parents or our peers walk it and we can relate to their experience. The unfamiliar is a scary place with great uncertainty. With a familiar course also comes the illusion that things will be easier somehow because we have an idea of what we can expect, so we believe we can handle it. There's no certainty in life and absolutely no easy road. There is only inspired versus dull; the choice is our own.

The question, "who are you to do this?" can apply to anything—really anything at all. In all honesty, that doubt has surfaced during the process of writing this book. But I relentlessly chose to continue subscribing wholeheartedly to the notion that I am as good as anybody to write it. A new holy communion among my mind, body, and true nature allowed me to safely pass by that brief brush of uncertainty unscathed.

It's true that you're never going to escape fearful moments. Worrisome thoughts can and will drift in and out of the mind freely, but the deep-seated emotions or established beliefs about yourself will determine if those thoughts are allowed to grow as weeds, blocking the passage to an inspiring life, which can ultimately spark the desire to comfort eat.

Imagine your physical self as a secret little garden. The mind is the threshold to where our energy has the ability to transform seeds of thoughts into real matter to be carried forth by way of actions and ultimately, habits. Each thought that comes into your mind can be either dismissed and deemed of ill importance, or it can be regarded as truth and be remembered and referenced at a later date. If your mind perceives it to be true, it will then allow it to physically become a part of you.

The mind is the library of stored information that we refer to as a resource in every single moment and in every decision we make. Each of our daily interactions and choices in this world are the direct result of the data we chose to keep locked up in there.

How we learn something

Chances are, if I ask you where you were when you first heard of the terrorist attacks on 9/11, you would be able to, in detail, describe to me where you were. Yet, if I asked you about any other arbitrary day that year, you wouldn't have a clue where you were or what you were doing. Am I right?

It appears that emotionally charged situations can lead us to create longer-lasting memories of the event. In other words, what gives our memories a fighting chance to survive in our mind is the degree to which they are accompanied by an emotion. The greater the emotional quotient, the greater the likelihood we remember the event. There is an incredible wisdom in evolution that allows for this design, as it increases our tendency to learn from our experience and gives us a greater chance of survival.

In recent years, the subject of neuroplasticity has gained growing popularity. There's no short and simple explanation that can describe this marvel to its true magnificence, but if you aren't yet familiar with it, allow me to briefly explain.

Your brain consists of grey matter and white matter. The grey matter contains billions of neurons and other cells of the central nervous system. Sensory information coming into the brain immediately gets divided into fragments and sent to various regions within the brain. When we learn new information, a neuron—called a presynaptic neuron—sends a neurotransmitter through what's called a synaptic cleft. This act sends a message to a receiving neuron named the postsynaptic neuron. Once the postsynaptic neuron receives the signal, it can either reject the information by turning itself off—a process referred to as inhibition—or it can deem it useful, allowing the signal to pass through. Through a process termed reuptake, the neurotransmitter is sent back to the first neuron. When learning takes place, the two neurons begin to form a path connecting to one another. Storing information is not just limited to two neurons; a whole heap of connections can be made simultaneously throughout many regions in the brain.

Some of our neurological connections are what researchers refer to as "experience-independent," for example, breathing or pumping blood through our veins. Rather, experience-dependent wiring is the stored information we gather through experience that we become conditioned to. While the experience-independent part of our brain is hardwired, the more flexible experience-dependent part of our brain is given a generous amount of space to download data based on experiences. Our brain is an incredibly adaptive little machine that is sensitive to the environment it finds itself in. This is why no two brains are wired alike, and why personal beliefs can vary drastically from person to person.

When we experience something (real or imagined) more than once—repeat our behaviours, learn a lesson, hear a judgment, or re-live a memory—the connection between the neurons becomes stronger. The intensity of the emotions that accompanies the experience is the measure by which the brain will deem its significance, allowing the connection to fasten more securely.

The degree to which something is a universal truth, and the weight and space it holds inside your mind, are not linked. With each repetition of thought, connecting neurons will fire together and wire together stronger, and the path between the two will grow larger. Imagine it like walking on a path. Each time you take that same path, it becomes a little more clearly paved. Eventually, it may become a road, and with enough traction over time, it could turn into a major highway. Your brain doesn't like to take the back streets; it prefers what it knows, and would rather run along the more efficient roads of the highways—it's a productive little machine. Everything we learn works this way.

Of course, the opposite is also true; use it or lose it very much applies in this case. Stories we stop running in our minds, events we give little significance to, or routines we stop executing, eventually fade away through a process called synaptic pruning, also referred to as forgetting. Synaptic pruning helps regulate efficiency and energy conservation. The less we use a pathway, the greater the chance it will begin to fade.

What's really important to note here is that experiencing an event repetitively isn't necessarily limited to our body's external border. Simply recalling a memory, and then re-living it inside your mind, is enough for your brain to recognize it as a repeated experience— the memory or belief is then granted a heftier block of real estate.

Two heavy influencers on what you pay attention to are your memories and emotions. For day-to-day decisions, your brain uses the data from previous experiences to determine what you pay attention to. So in other words, our internal emotions govern most of what we see in the outside world.

The existing belief about yourself and your life is a huge factor in determining what you will continue to see and experience. If there is a running unconscious emotion that has flooded your mind and body, it prohibits you from believing you have just as much value as everyone else; it hinders you from seeing a future of anything greater. It will never grant you the permission to make decisions from a place of love for yourself, either.

Your emotions can be thought of as energy in motion. They consist of matter, and they have the ability to get stronger. Imagine your garden for a moment, and picture yourself as the one who provides the instructions and blueprints to a gardener who does its upkeep. The gardener is your subconscious mind that's been heavily programmed through your emotions and experiences. You have conscious control of your thoughts and therefore, you ultimately get to decide if you want to live among weeds or if you want to commit to systematically pruning each old emotion while sowing new, loving, compassionate seeds.

Here's the thing... No one is coming to save you. Nobody is coming. I cried the first time I realized that— like a baby. No event, no person, no monetary gain, no special diet, no job, and certainly no knight in shining armour was coming to save me, and that is the magical moment where something shifted inside of me.

Faith: Complete trust or confidence in someone or something.

Several years ago, the universe sent a series of events my way, which were the catalysts that catapulted me into a completely new direction and environment. Overnight, there was a drastic change in my environment that I had been surviving in for the preceding six years. I remember my mind flooding with reasons why I may not have had the ability to lead this new life, an endless stream of reasons why I could potentially fail. Fortunately, failure was not an option. I simply wasn't going to crumble and die. I had no plan and so out of desperation, I prayed, "Please, universe or divine power or whatever you are, please tell me what to do. Just tell me the next step I should take. I am not asking for anything except for guidance. Amen."

As I opened my eyes, the word FAITH appeared in front of me, barely visible, suspended in mid-air. *Okay, that's something, I suppose,* I thought to myself. *Not only am I completely lost, but now I am seeing things too; this should be good.* I grabbed a Sharpie pen that happened to be sitting next to me and I wrote the word out on my left hand, in the same bold, capital, block letters, just as they appeared in the vision.

What was I supposed to do with this word? What was I meant to have faith in? As the child growing up who used to take apart all the electronic things in our house just to see how they worked and where it all started, I had a little trouble just simply having faith. Nevertheless, I was going to give it a try. I mean, these were letters suspended in space; that almost never happens.

No more than a day later, I spotted this word, etched in a little, silver pendant in the jewellery case of a local department store. Obviously, I was going to buy it; I mean, who wouldn't? Suspended letters in space have now magically appeared before me in real matter. You could say I wore it religiously. On days when I would feel lost, catching the necklace in my reflection as I passed a mirror always gave me a tiny dose of strength. The constant reminder of the word FAITH gave me the ability to not only keep looking forward, but to also walk away from my past and let go of it with a little bit of grace.

The thing about faith is that it works better when you know what you have faith in.

When I was growing up, my stepfather introduced my sister and me to religion. At the time, learning, understanding, and accepting everything he taught us was something I needed to adapt to in order to survive in my environment. My stepfather was our perceived lifeline in that time and space. He provided for my family; in addition, my mother found some security in his intelligence, drive, and social status and consequently, so did I. He also believed in the idea of "spare the rod, spoil the child," and I wasn't a huge fan of the rod, so the few questions I had about that faith I kept to myself, burying them deep in the depths of my mind. I was certainly not going to allow those thoughts to grow. Doing this was imperative to my survival—not that I connected all this at the time. The stories and imagery made just enough sense to me that I could convince all the cells in my body that they were true—survival of the fittest thoughts, as I like to call it. Confidence in these perceived facts, and this trust in something outside of me, moulded much of who I was in grade school.

Like all things in life, changes occurred and, in my late teens, ignoring those little questions I had about organized religion no longer suited me. Moreover, my new habitat had the right conditions that allowed those questions, thoughts, or seeds in my mind to grow. As they grew, I adapted to the idea that my beliefs just weren't working for me anymore. I grew to describe myself as "spiritual, but not religious." This was another beneficial adaptation to my thoughts, because it allowed me to connect to my next lifeline.

At the age of 22, I met someone. I found him truly fascinating; we shared many of the same ideas about the world, and we had an incredible ability to teach each other things. This man, my perceived soulmate at the time, was my best friend; he was also educated, had confidence in his future direction, came from a good family, and he took care of me in many of the same ways my stepfather did; so I married him. I loved him dearly, but a lot of the confidence I displayed during this time was a result of a sense of security we gave one another.

The two of us were a force to be reckoned with. We were a power couple, to say the least. He was a doctor, and taught me all about health and wellness, an area which I'd always had a keen interest in. He displayed so many traits that I perceived were missing or under-developed within me, and I am certain he felt exactly the same way about me. We both had a false sense of wholeness, and all we needed was each other to have the confidence to face the world.

I now had an increased sense of confidence, and I felt it was time for me to go back to school and learn about an area that had always intrigued me. After a considerable amount of self-debate about whether I could actually do it, I decided it was worth the investment and I began nutritional studies. This was a decision I would have never allowed myself to make had I been on my own, because I didn't believe I could do it alone. I only granted myself the permission to move forward because I believed I had this amazing support system in my husband, who I had convinced myself was somehow more intelligent than I was. I was assured that it would only be through his help that I would make it through the years.

As it turned out, I didn't need any outside help. I absorbed the information like a sponge. It was near the end of my first semester when I first learned there was an undeniable link between nutrition and mental wellbeing. It was then I knew exactly what I wanted to do with my life. I went to my husband and shared my dreams to continue studying, eventually combining nutrition with alternate therapies so I could find a path to help people overcome emotional eating. His reaction was not one I had expected, and only two days later I found out exactly why. For the previous three weeks, he had been preparing to leave me—and he did just that.

"I don't love you anymore."

This is the event that led me to that faith necklace. I was desperate to find faith in something, and despite the fact that I couldn't describe what I was having faith in, I continued to have it. Even though there were days when I didn't even want to bother to wake up, I continually got up every morning as early as 4:30 a.m. for my morning workouts, worked 16-hour days to save money for my tuition, and continued my studies, eventually completing the program with honours.

I was a heartbroken, insecure, single female, armed with only faith in who knows what, and a million fearful thoughts that carried so much weight in my decisions. Something inside told me incessantly that it was now time to face all of my fears. This included jumping off a bridge (of course, attached to a bungee cord). With each fear I faced and with each passing day, my self-assurance started to grow. But along the journey, more fears continued to emerge. I started to realize that the hardest step was always taking that initial leap. I found this revealing because that is the moment when I was still standing securely, and technically still safe. Once I made the jump, it wasn't nearly as frightening as I had imagined it would be.

It was about 18 months after my separation when I met a girl randomly on the street. She, for no apparent reason, began telling me about her recent separation. I could feel her pain with every fibre of my being. This girl was just like me, only a year earlier. I explained the story of my faith necklace and as tears filled her eyes, she said to me, "My friends don't understand what I am going through. I think you will be the one to help me. I must have met you for a reason." I knew then that telling her the story of my faith necklace was not enough, and what I really needed to do was give her the experience too. So I took off my necklace and tied it around her neck. The two of us instantly burst into tears. It was without a doubt the right thing to do, but the moment I saw it suspended around her neck, I realized I had just given my external power source away.

Days later, I randomly found another pendant online, one that really resonated with me at the time. The script showed the quote, "Be the change you wish to see in the world." Over the quote was a picture of what appeared to be a mustard seed plant. I bought the pendant but had no idea what a mustard seed plant represented. One day, out of sheer boredom, I typed in the search engine "images of mustard seed plants," and what I found blew me away—a collection of images with the plant and the word FAITH. I had no idea these two things could be linked. As it turns out there is a Scripture that reads, "If you have faith as small as a mustard seed, you can say to this mountain, 'Move from here to there,' and it will move. Nothing will be impossible for you." (Matthew 17:20)

Facing my anxieties, trying to live by "Be the change you wish to see in the world," exercising the idea of having faith as small as a mustard seed, were the perfect combination of nutrients my brain needed to produce the thoughts that grew to new beliefs about myself. I finally granted myself permission to conceive the idea that the only power source I could eternally keep faith in was myself.

From that moment forward, I made the decision that only thoughts that were from a place of love for myself were allowed to live and grow and flourish inside my mind.

We will come back to this story…

51

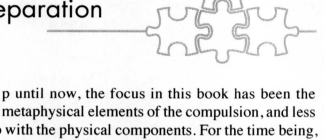

CHAPTER 5
Preparation

U p until now, the focus in this book has been the metaphysical elements of the compulsion, and less to do with the physical components. For the time being, we are going to hold our metaphysical train of thought and jump over to address the physical.

Anyone who says that a food addiction is all in the mind has not felt its ill effects on the body.

What incredibly addictive substance is a hard, white, crystal-like structure that rots your teeth and gets you hooked through invoking a feeling of euphoria triggered by dopamine in your brain?

If you didn't know better from the title of this book and what you've already read, then you could easily mistake this for crack cocaine. But yes, of course, I am referring in this case to sugar.

We are biologically wired to desire sweet foods because they deliver immediate energy and storage for potential future famine—which was often a reality for our ancestors. In addition, we have a similar eagerness for foods high in fat. Today, in developed countries, scarcity of food is no longer a prevailing issue; indeed, we are blessed with a feast almost everywhere we go. But the part of our brain that regulates hunger and appetite have yet to catch up with this abundance. The food industry is in the business of engineering artificial energy-dense foods that are designed with one main goal in mind—to play on our desires and ensure we keep coming back for more. These foods, in my opinion, should not even be classified as food at all because they often provide little to no nourishment, and resemble a drug more than actual food. These engineered, food-like substances are being deliberately created to target the primal part of our brain so that we find them irresistible.

A sugar addiction is more common than the masses would like to concede. Below is an idea of what a typical meal plan would be like for someone who, with great conviction, tries to convince me that they don't have a sugar addiction.

- Morning: coffee with sugar with a low-fat muffin baked with sugar, or a bowl of oatmeal with brown sugar.
- Mid-day: veggie snack, dipped in a sugary salad dressing.
- Lunch: a cup of liquid sugar (soft drink or juice) to wash down two slices of bread (baked with sugar) stuffed with some kind of luncheon meat containing sugar.
- Dinner: something sprinkled, dipped, coated, or marinated in sugar, with a side of something else sprinkled, dipped, coated, or marinated in sugar, and don't forget the soft drink.
- Dessert: I think it's safe to assume there is going to be some sugar.

There are a ton of variables that lead to the craving of sugar, but one very common and perhaps the easiest to manage is low blood sugar. When your blood glucose gets low, your brain sends some very powerful and impossible to resist signals for you to quickly eat something. So, we do exactly that. We tend to choose from the above meals, or something like them. Some people might even reach for something worse, like a donut or a cookie. These all provide too much of a "good thing." Your blood doesn't need all that glucose at once. In fact, if it's not a naturally occurring sugar in a whole food, then your body doesn't need it at all. The best thing I ever did for myself was to cut refined sugar out of my life completely, and I highly recommend that for everybody.

Your blood only needs a very small amount of glucose at a time. The glucose level that defines hypoglycaemia (low blood sugar) varies slightly from person to person, but about a teaspoon of glucose in your blood is ideal; even a few grams of extra sugar in your bloodstream can be life-threatening. After eating a sugary or high-carbohydrate meal, we have an excessive and dangerously high level of sugar in our bloodstream. Once your body senses this alarming supply of sugar in the blood, it signals your pancreas to release insulin.

Insulin is also known as the fat-storing stress hormone. Insulin comes to your rescue and saves you from what you just ate. Our bodies are really spectacular this way. They respond very quickly in this emergency circumstance. But of course, insulin rushes in and takes the toxic dose of sugar from your blood and stores it as fat. What's even more exciting is, when all that insulin is released during this emergency state, it can take from your blood most, if not all, of the sugar you just ate. And that takes you right back to where you started before you ate. Now you have low blood sugar again. Low blood glucose, or hypoglycaemia, is an equally dangerous state to high blood sugar or hyperglycaemia.

Now the hypoglycaemic state has got your brain sending those very familiar and powerful signals, inducing cravings that are impossible to refrain from. What typically happens at this stage is we find it an impossible task to resist that sugar-filled mid-day snack and thus, the cycle goes on for the rest of the day.

Think about it like this—if you were to start your day with a huge hit of crack cocaine, then chances are you'd be hitting that crack pipe all day. It's important to understand that the sugar train works much the same.

They often call breakfast the most important meal of the day for many reasons, but I believe one of the most important reasons—as it relates to food addiction—is breakfast's ability to set the stage for blood sugar control for the rest of the day. A heavy carbohydrate breakfast can, and will, have you spending the entire day in either a state of high or low blood sugar.

Why cravings are so powerful during states of hypoglycaemia.

Being a nutritionist can sometimes be incredibly frustrating, especially when it comes to the subject of shedding weight. When passing suggestions to clients, I often get cut off before I can offer any real guidance. "I already know what I need to do," they proclaim, generally followed with an, "I just have to do it."

In all honesty, I am aware that you have an idea of what you should be eating. Everyone and their dog knows that if you quit eating dessert and you start eating kale, then you are likely to shed weight. What it takes to eat clean is really no big secret these days. Those who state that they already know what to do are often no different than the vast majority.

To date, I have yet to hear anyone say to me, "My new year's resolution this year is to be as unhealthy as possible. Starting Monday morning, I am going to do whatever it takes to quit the gym, I'm going to hire a trainer and he is going to force me to binge eat on fast food, ice cream, and chips." With that in mind, it's fairly safe to assume that most people really do want to be fitter and healthier. So if we all want to be in great shape and we already know what it takes to be healthier, why then aren't we all successfully doing it?

The answer is not in the what, but in the why.

Knowing what not to eat doesn't address or defeat the most deliciously evil part of the battle—the insidious food cravings!

One major catalyst for food cravings is that your brain is extremely selfish.

During fasting or starvation, all of the organs in your body will make adjustments to conserve energy. They can actually shrink in size to adapt to the current situation, except for your brain, of course. The brain is the most demanding organ of the body. It puts its needs first and serves itself first. The brain's main source of fuel is glucose (sugar), and it also happens to be the primary consumer of glucose. At only 2 percent of the total body weight, the brain uses a whopping 20 percent or so of the body's energy, give or take about 500k cal/

day. During acute mental stress, the energy supply to the human brain increases by about 12 percent.

Moreover, the brain doesn't have much of an energy storing system. For that, the brain depends on the body. This is referred to as "energy on demand." When the brain needs energy and the blood stores are low, it takes it from the energy stores (fat stores) of the body, turning the fat into glucose and using it as fuel; it's an ingenious design. When the body's stores eventually run out, it will demand it from the external environment (food). As clever as this design may be, there can be a glitch in this system if there is a defect in the control systems of the brain. Extreme stress, advertising from sweets (which we are constantly exposed to), and conditioning of eating behaviour can be among the factors leading to these defects. So, instead of using the body's energy store for glucose, it demands it directly from food. This surplus of energy can accumulate, leading to increased fat stores in the body. But your selfish brain doesn't mind, because it is temporarily happy, and that is its priority! This phenomenon is known as "The Selfish Brain Theory."

If you repetitively satisfy your low blood sugar with junk food, you give your subconscious mind positive reinforcement that these foods will relatively quickly give your brain what it wants, and lots of it, at that. Each time you repeat this behaviour, you strengthen the synaptic connections in your brain. The repetition reaffirms the routine within the body. At this stage, binge eating becomes a wickedly powerful and dangerously impulsive habit that the body plays out without much conscious instruction from the mind. When the body becomes programmed to think faster than the conscious mind, that habit becomes an addiction, leaving even the strongest mind feeling like a hopeless prisoner repeatedly surrendering their conscious mind's goals and needs.

Many people say, "But I don't crave sugar; I lean toward salty or savoury." With all due respect, if you truly believe that, you are fooling yourself. What's more, many of those salty and savoury treats also contain sugar. Even those who think they aren't addicted to sugar often are. I highly recommend, for a week, to try going off all sugars and sweeteners, to fully have a grasp at how addictive this substance truly is. A sugar addiction is viciously powerful, and I believe is far more prevalent in society than we are prepared to accept. Nonetheless, if your cravings tend to be for salty or savoury things, then this is still largely in part due to the selfish brain theory.

The brain gets its nutrients from the blood, passing the blood-brain barrier via a special insulin-independent transport system. When your blood pressure gets low, the blood flow to your brain decreases. You can imagine that this would make your very selfish brain exceedingly angry. It has very cleverly learned from past experience that where salt goes, water goes. In other words, salt pulls fluid into your blood vessels, expanding them and making it easier for your heart to pump blood to your brain. Our little brain is quite a bit savvier than we give it credit for. Again, every time you repeat this behaviour, you reinforce your brain to behave in the same manner the next time there are similar circumstances. This is in special thanks to our friend, neuroplasticity.

Here's the kicker—postprandial hypotension is low blood pressure that comes a couple hours after a meal, and is related to the surplus of glucose in a carbohydrate meal, to the insulin spike, and to the sugar crash that follows this spike. A sugar crash can be induced by caffeine, desserts, or simply a heavy carbohydrate meal. This can explain why sweet cravings are often followed by ravenous salt cravings; your brain knows what's coming. In some instances, it can get really sly and demand both at the same time. Next thing you know, you are eating ice cream straight out of the tub, only to take breaks to shove a handful of pretzels down your face. I know it may be hard to believe, but you are not the only one who has done that, and now you have some understanding of why you have.

The food industry has used this information to their advantage by cleverly designing foods that will cause us to reach what is known as the bliss point. In the formulation of engineered food-like products, the bliss point is the amount of and combinations of ingredients such as sugar, salt, and fat that optimises palatability.

So what can be done to abate this mess?

I can't stress the importance enough of being kind to yourself when and if you do fall off the wagon. Don't panic, and please don't beat yourself up over it. Blame, shame, guilt, and anger only give way to comfort eating, thus turning your "treat" into a guilty pleasure. We were all doomed by the introduction of the word "treat" (I'm not sure whose bright idea that was, but I propose we all change the meaning of that word in our vocabulary).

59

Anytime you have one of these negative thoughts, you release a neurochemical that leads you to feel that thought throughout the body; we call these feelings emotions. Replaying that thought over and over in your mind repeats the release of these hormones and other chemicals in your brain and body. Over time, with thoughts alone, you have the ability to cause a self-induced chemical imbalance that affects your mood, personality, and ultimately, your self-medicating habits.

Have you ever wondered why you don't emotionally eat when you are happy? Happy thoughts can release the neurotransmitter serotonin. Serotonin is an appetite suppressant. Your mood, your thoughts, and your hormonal state have supremacy over your appetite, which is why I have chosen to focus on these areas in later chapters. If you happen to relapse, forgiving yourself immediately and then moving forward without obsessing over your recent decisions are more crucial to your recovery than you might initially conceive.

Instead of beating yourself up over it, make a new choice this time, and let go. What's done is done, and what matters now is breaking the rest of the pattern. Go back up to the list you wrote in the chapter on surrogacy, then pick something on that list that would best recede your guilty feelings. Call friends, do yoga, make love, paint, watch a comedy, take a bath, or do anything that works for you. Think of "raindrops on roses and whiskers on kittens" if that lifts your spirits—just do anything but more sulking and eating!

How to balance blood sugar

- Don't let your blood glucose levels drop to dangerously low levels. If you are trying to adopt new eating habits, then make sure you are always prepared with a wholesome snack that is ready to eat when you get hungry. Don't let yourself get caught with low blood sugar, and with nothing healthy that's ready and available for you to eat. We have become familiar with willpower and how unimpressively it performs during hypoglycaemic states. Don't risk it, and for heaven's sake, eat when you feel hungry, because you won't stand a chance once you've hit starving.

- Caffeine, heavy carbohydrate meals, starving oneself, and stress can lead to fluctuating hyper and hypoglycaemia. Do whatever it takes to reduce or eliminate these things in your life. To give yourself a fighting chance, don't start your morning with processed sugar.

- Processed or refined foods (white sugar, sweeteners, white breads, pastas, packaged foods, etc.) are stripped of their beneficial fibre, causing rapid spikes to your body glucose level, invariably leading to increased insulin release. Fruit is a nutritious way to quickly raise blood sugar. A half-cup of fresh fruit (ex., grapefruit or berries) before you eat any meal can bring your blood sugar to a safe level, which may reduce cravings or overeating during meals. It can quite possibly help you make better food choices for the duration of your day. Unrefined whole foods like fruits and vegetables are high in fibre, which slows down the release of glucose into your bloodstream, helping your blood sugar stay steady throughout the day.

- It's important to refrain from baked goods and heavy, starchy, or refined carbs, at all times of the day, especially at breakfast. Sure, you're more likely to burn off these early morning calories, but you're also be more likely to ride the sugar-coaster all day. While adopting new eating patterns, it's essential to remember that vegetables are a safe bet, and they are loaded with nutrition that can help balance the entire body.

- If you need additional help devising your own meal plan that helps control blood glucose levels, then find a nutritionist in your local area who has a philosophy that resonates with yours. Alternatively, you could follow the guidelines in my program "The Eating Enigma: 90 days to transform your relationship with food," which is available for purchase at www.mariaayne.com.

- To give yourself a fighting chance, don't keep garbage in the house! If you are stressed, tired, hungry, or you are in the middle of a bout of willpower fatigue, and treats are right there staring you dead in the eye, then you will eat them—you are only human. Why set yourself up for failure? Understand your limitations and reduce the temptations from your home, at work, and the other most common environments you find yourself in. Remember that all it takes is a cue in your environment to set off the subconscious program of seeking the reward. If the cue is a box filled with donuts, then it's in your best interest that you don't keep that cue sitting in your fridge.

- If your partner or housemate isn't on board with your food revolution, and he or she insists on keeping treats in and around the house, then perhaps just try changing the location of the unhealthy food. Breaking patterns is key! Replace everything that was in your usual junk-filled pantry with healthy alternatives, or even encouraging notes and pictures of your goals. The last thing you need is a bunch of reminders of your old habits just lying around taunting you in your own home.

- Chewing your food thoroughly before you swallow it is vastly underrated. The first stage of digestion happens in your mouth. Chewing not only helps break down the food while it is in your mouth, it also sends signals to your stomach that food is coming. These signals allow your digestive system to release the appropriate enzymes it needs in order to digest that particular food. For example, protein needs protease to be broken down, carbohydrates need amylase, and fats require lipase. Our body is so much more amazing than we give it credit for. Failing to chew slows down and disrupts the digestive processes. Your selfish brain doesn't have the patience for slow; you don't want to make it angry, do you?

- And finally, of course, there is the wonderful world of exercise, which in my opinion, deserves novels of its own. But for the sake of giving you as much information as possible, I will briefly touch on the topic. Physical exercise can help lower blood glucose in the short-term because when your muscles contract during activity, it stimulates another mechanism that is completely separate from insulin. This mechanism allows your cells to take up glucose and use it for energy in the absence of insulin.

Nutritional Deficiencies

Apart from low blood sugar, dysfunctional eating can lead to nutritional shortages in the body, and those deficiencies can absolutely affect your food choices. They also hold the power to negatively affect your mood—which greatly influences food cravings.

- Chocoholic: A chocoholic is a person who craves or compulsively consumes chocolate. "Chocoholism" is quite common. In studies of food cravings, chocolate and chocolate confectioneries almost always top the list of foods people say they crave. According to WebMD, women are especially vulnerable to having this behavior.

Chocolate is an addiction so powerful it has earned its way into dictionary.com and wikipedia.org. Well played, chocolate; well played. But what brings this rich chocolate delight to the top of everyone's list of foods they crave? What is in this little bean that has led so many people, especially women, to be so vulnerable? It can't be the taste alone. In all honesty, raw cacao bean has got to be one of the most offensive things I have ever tasted. Some might argue that when working with the right accomplices—sugar and fat—it tastes quite divine, but so does everything else, short of mud. When doing a comparison on just taste, I might even say I prefer vanilla; but I've never really craved a vanilla cake. In fact, according to my sources—dictionary. com and wikipedia.org—vanillaholic isn't even a word, despite vanilla being the secret weapon in so many desserts. The chocolate puzzle must have another layer.

I will refer to that layer as magnesium.

Magnesium is an essential mineral, meaning we need it to survive. We exhaust our body's reserves more rapidly in times of stress, fatigue, physical exertion, and of course, during the female menstrual cycle. Some dietary sources of magnesium include spices, nuts, cereals, dark leafy green vegetables, and cacao.

You could argue that, if chocolate is on that list, then it must be healthy. While the philosophy on the cacao bean and nutrition wavers depending on the nutritionist, the kind of chocolate confectionery you crave when you are stressed is pretty unanimously agreed by all experts to be a nutritional villain.

The false thought pattern that "I am craving it, so my body must need it" falls a little short here, as most people don't crave many of those other foods on that list the way they do chocolate, yet some of them are more abundant sources of magnesium. Ah, yet another layer to this addictive thriller.

This layer can also be known as zinc.

Low zinc is a common mineral deficiency, and zinc happens to be used up more rapidly in the body when we consume and metabolize sweet treats. Some of the first signs of a zinc deficiency include a reduced sense of smell, loss of appetite, and how we taste food. All of these factors make you less likely to reach for spinach when magnesium stores are low and more likely to reach for a more powerful sensation, like a hit of sweetened chocolate. The taste of nuts and cereals just don't have quite the same bite as that dark bean.

It's a vicious little spiral, as each time we succumb to the compulsion to reach for our favourite chocolate dessert, we simultaneously further create another deficiency that leads us to prefer to reach for that same chocolate dessert next time around and less likely to want anything to do with the much healthier options. What's worse is, it is often those with powerful food cravings who are also the notorious perpetual dieters, adding yet another portion to the recipe for the zinc deficiency disaster. Those who restrict food intake are the most vulnerable to this compounding wreck. Restricting calories, skipping meals, and cutting off certain food sources are among the main culprits to so many nutritional deficiencies in first world countries. Zinc is right there at the top of the mineral deficiency list. Although no less wicked than any other nutritional deficiency, the absence of any essential nutrient can devastate the body.

I can't express enough concern when it comes to quick and fast fad diets, as many people don't really understand what the long-term consequences are. Often these fads will initially produce some desirable results, but that doesn't mean they will continue to. Besides that, the consequences to your body could be very difficult to undo.

There is no diet as impressive as the one that Mother Nature sets for us. There is no google search quite as clever at constructing a meal plan as she is. Eat seasonal, eat local, eat organic, eat whole foods, eat a variety, eat mindfully, and eat only when you are hungry.

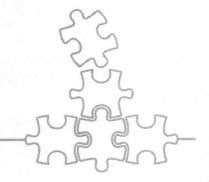

CHAPTER 6

Population

<u>Your Personal Support System</u>

I t's estimated that you have about 100 trillion bacteria making up one universal ecosystem. These bacteria are thought to outnumber your human cells 10:1, and a considerable amount of these creatures reside in your gut. There is a tiny ecosystem within your gut that could also be contributing a significant vote when it comes to your ultimate choices at mealtime.

Before you put me in a straightjacket for suggesting that single-celled organisms might be controlling your thoughts, and you protest, "They can't do that!" let me tell you a few things they can do…

Evolve

While your genetic code takes a human lifetime to be passed down to the next generation, these tiny microbes only take hours to do the same. Their ability to reproduce so fast also increases their opportunities to evolve as rapidly as our external environment is changing. For millions of years they have been co-evolving alongside animals, just as they are continuing to do on us. Their survival is partly dependant on us, and they also return the favour by contributing to our existence.

When one of these critters living on our bodies does something that we like or that we feel benefits us, we call them "good bacteria." And when they do something we don't like or cause our bodies to respond in an undesirable manner, we call them "bad bacteria."

What are a few things they do that we like and don't like?

Well, for starters, they can help us digest our food. You may be wondering just how much impact they can possibly make on digestion, and the answer may surprise you. Cows, who eat a grass diet, don't actually have much of an ability to get any nutrition from the grass on their own. Instead, they depend on the bugs living in their four-chambered stomach to produce the enzymes they need to digest this high-fibre diet. I know what you are thinking; "But we aren't cows." While that's a fantastic observation, just know that they make a similar contribution for us as well.

Synthesize Vitamins

We've known for a long time now that the bacteria in our gut also produce many vitamins that are essential to maintaining good health. For example, vitamin k, which is an essential nutrient needed for blood clotting, is produced by the bacteria in our gut. Without this vitamin, you could bleed to death from a tiny cut. There is also increasing attention towards the link between a lack of vitamin k and inflammatory bowel disease. So, they digest our food and produce vitamins we need to survive. So far, these pests aren't so bad.

Until, of course, you're standing at the checkout aisle of your local grocery store and just next to you is the most gorgeous human you've ever seen. You can't even believe your luck as you begin to flirt with each other. Then suddenly, oh no, is that gas? You knew you shouldn't have had that dairy in your latte this morning! As a bead of sweat drips down your face you think, *Maybe I can hold…* Oh, there it goes, and it's a stinker. The smell wafts through the store while all eyes turn on you. You look back and your dream man or woman has already bee-lined it straight out the door and into their car where they are safe from your obnoxious fumes. You can thank your gut bacteria for that chemical warfare too.

Besides toxic chemicals, they can release hormones as well, and they have a direct route from the gut to the brain through the vagus nerve. Hormones are the almighty chemicals that lead to all kinds of reactions within the body. As we have already learned, our emotions are governed by these hormones. For instance, dopamine makes you feel motivated; serotonin can lead to euphoria and reduced appetite; and then there are others, such as the hormone leptin, which is released by the lining of your stomach when your stomach has been filled. Leptin travels to your brain, signaling that you are full and you should stop eating. Without leptin, you would never feel satisfied. You would never know you were full, and you would continue to eat everything in sight. To complicate matters a little bit, it's now known that bacteria can interfere with hormones, one of those said hormones being leptin. Studies have also confirmed that microbiota affects anxiety by influencing brain neurochemistry.

With thousands of different species of bacteria inhabiting your body and calling it their home, each of these species is fighting one another for the greatest portion of real estate and for their chance to dominate. Their desire to let another cross their respective borders seems to be even less tolerant than ours; each one is doing what it takes to survive and to reproduce as fast as they can — which is at a forcible speed. All these passengers are at an ongoing dinner party while we are playing the host. They eat what we serve them, and what we feed these little critters heavily influences which ones get to win the war. Unfortunately, the diet each species needs to thrive is not all alike. The choices we make at each and every meal determines which species get a fighting chance and which ones are at a major disadvantage.

When you put together all these facts about these little guys, the notion that they might be influencing your food cravings becomes a little easier to digest.

Since our gut bacteria are anaerobic (live in the absence of air, or free from oxygen), they have been exceptionally difficult to study up until recently. As a result, very little has been understood of their influence on our health. New research techniques have made the impossible possible, and we are now gaining insight about their complex symbiotic relationship with our health. Researchers are investigating the link between specific gut flora profiles and health outcomes by looking for associations with specific health characteristics and those specific gut flora profiles. Researchers

71

have found a strong link between diversity of gut bacteria and mind-altering effects on our behaviour.

Ultimately, you have the final say on whether or not you give in to your food cravings. Each and every one of your food choices casts a vote on their election. Research shows that the diversity in our gut can drastically change in a matter of a few days with a new diet. A high-fibre, plant-based diet will lead to greater numbers of some species, while a diet low in fibre and richer in meat sources could lead you to house a whole other group. On the same note, a highly refined junk-food diet has the capacity to sway the power towards a whole other group.

It is likely that the foods you are accustomed to eating are the exact foods the predominant species in your gut need to continue to survive, and that is why you continue to crave them. For billions of years, if bacteria have shown us one thing at all, it is that they will do absolutely whatever they need to do to survive. These microbes are under no moral obligation to play fair, and the fact that you want to get beach-body ready ranks a whopping zero on their priority list.

When you eat real food that is given to you by Mother Nature, it shows that over time you actually start to prefer this lifestyle and your body learns to adapt to crave these whole foods. This may be heavily influenced by a change in your gut bacteria that are sending you signals to ensure you maintain this new meal plan, so that they can continue to monopolize.

Introducing fermented foods into your diet can help you maintain the diversity in your gut that is needed to keep a balanced ecosystem. This diversity ensures that organisms, such as candida, don't grow in such numbers that they become out of control. The body is meant to have candida, but the problems begin to arise when the body lacks other microbes that help keep candida from over-colonizing. Candida feeds on sugar and relies on you for its supply. A diet high in refined sugars and artificial sweeteners, combined with low diversity of the other microbes needed to keep it at bay, leads to overgrowth, and many undesirable symptoms throughout the body.

You have an intricate world inside you, filled with microorganisms that have the ability to assist you on your healing journey, but their survival is dependent on the choices you make at every meal. You must keep them in mind; you want their support. Believe me when I say, their support matters.

Your External Support System

We, by our true nature, are pack animals. We need to belong to a community to feel safe. We were never the strongest species in the wild—we only sustained strength in numbers. With the development of our pre-frontal cortex, we are able to moderate social behaviour and orchestrate our thoughts and actions in harmony with personal goals. We have developed a level of communication so complex that it enabled us to pass information down to our offspring more effectively than any other species. By building on what our ancestors have taught us and by working together as part of a greater community, we have increased our chances of survival, and our adaptability to our environment. It was through this communication that we were able to build tools, orchestrate strategies, and make the necessary advancements in technology to propel us forward.

The yearning to belong is innate within the human species because it is paramount to our survival. It is in this community, and through connecting with one another, that we feel the most protected. From an evolutionary standpoint, belonging is a deep-seated need, because it meant that you were somewhat guarded against the dangers of the outside world; being alone made you feel vulnerable and exposed to great and real risk.

We feel uncomfortable at our core when we have to go to an event alone because we have no sense of security or familiarity. A familiar person by your side gives you a sense of assurance; oxytocin is the powerful chemical that is responsible for this social bonding. The release of oxytocin gives us that warm and fuzzy feeling we get inside when we fall in love. Being part of a team makes us feel good inside. Oxytocin is released in a number of ways: through physical touch, childbirth, and acts of service to a community.

Giving your time and energy for the benefit of humanity and receiving support from the society generates a feeling of love through the effects of oxytocin (also known as the hormone of love). Simply witnessing an act of service has the ability to release oxytocin. Physical touch strengthens our bonds. Cuddling releases large amounts of oxytocin, and mothers get a huge surge of oxytocin at childbirth — safeguarding their bond with their offspring.

A human baby would not survive without someone to care for it. The human brain — when fully developed — is too large to safely pass through the birth canal, so unlike other mammals, a great portion of our neurological development takes place in the years following birth.

We are hopeless in this world without each other; unity is a biological need.

We live in a society now where we are told we need to learn to be comfortable with being alone. Some of us live alone; we eat alone, and we often work at a goal alone, which by our very design is meant to make us feel extremely uncomfortable. Many of us live in homes with other people but are disconnected because we lead completely separate lives.

We feel like we will be shunned if we talk to someone about these unsettling feelings we are having. Longing for love has been misinterpreted and labeled as "needy." We have this distorted sense of reality that if we own more possessions than those who are less fortunate than us, we should always feel happy. Feeling negative implies that we are ungrateful for our blessings, and nobody wants to be labeled as ungrateful or needy, so instead of reaching out for support, which would serve as the antidote, we make the choice to retreat into ourselves.

The absence of human connection, of belonging to a tribe, and of being of service to each other, deprives us of that much-needed oxytocin. There is increased attention toward oxytocin for its potential to inhibit addictive behavior. Researchers theorise that it's very difficult to become addicted to something when we have our desired levels of oxytocin, so this "love hormone" has been spotlighted as a potential treatment for addictions. In other words, love might very well be the key to set us free.

There is a famous study conducted on rats that transformed the way we view addiction. 'Rat Park' was a study done in the late 1970s by psychologist Bruce K. Alexander and his colleagues at Simon Fraser University in British Columbia, Canada. Alexander found that caged rats who were isolated, when given the choice to drink plain water or water laced with morphine, chose the latter option, in contrast to rats that were exposed to an enriched environment with other rats; they significantly preferred to drink plain water.

Social acceptance is precious to us as a species. In fact, it is so valuable that we have become obsessed with thoughts of what people think of us, because rejection means we could be ostracized and cast out from society. Getting along with one another, following the rules, and mimicking our peers is a brilliant survival tactic.

A great problem can emerge when the traditions of our tribe and the habits we have adopted from our clan no longer suit us. An inner conflict arises when we try and adopt opposing traditions to the ones held by those in our fellowship; we are risking the very emotional contracts that keep us feeling safe and loved. Shedding old skin and reinventing ourselves puts us at risk of our greatest fear—being alone.

We no longer live in a time when we are isolated from other communities. We are exposed to new beliefs and radically opposing traditions on a daily basis, some of which we find highly intriguing. Our minds are being pried open as we are exposed to novel ideas and endless streams of possibilities, but out of the fear of judgment, we slam the doors closed to many of these possibilities. The result is a gap between what we want for ourselves, and what our tribe envisions for us. We can become paralysed with fear to adopt a new lifestyle if it isn't in accordance with the values of the crowd. A violent internal battle between the need to fit in and the desire to walk our own path erupts.

It's easy to understand then, how we might sabotage our goals at the expense of fitting in.

There is a truism that states "you are an average of the people you spend the most time with." We have a tendency to emulate the actions and download the beliefs of those we surround ourselves with.

Our relationships require us to understand other perspectives while dealing with a long list of emotions. Language is imprecise and therefore unreliable, so we must also rely on our ability to tune in to those subtle shifts in tone of voice, and to be acutely aware of the muted vocabulary of body language. Mirror neurons are responsible for what has been dubbed *emotional empathy*, enabling us to connect with those around us by helping us understand how the other person is feeling.

Mirror neurons are a primate phenomenon discovered by a team of neurophysiologists at the University of Parma in Italy in the 1980s. Neurophysiologists Giacomo Rizzolatti, Giuseppe Di Pellegrino, Luciano Fadiga, Leonardo Fogassi, and Vittorio Gallese conducted an experiment that led to a fascinating discovery. During each experiment they permitted their subject, a monkey, to reach for food, as they recorded a single neuron's response to the certain movements related to reaching for its food. What they discovered was that when one of the researchers moved his arm, neurons in the brain of the monkey would respond in the same location as when the monkey moved his own arm. They found these specific neurons fired both when the monkey watched a person picking up a piece of food, as well as when the monkey itself picked up the food. This observation provides an explanation for why we can find ourselves yawning when we witness someone else yawning.

Researchers found that mirroring neurons are greatly influential in the development of language, and in our inclination to imitate those who surround us. By simply observing someone, we are able to share in what they are feeling. We can have a strong gut feeling if something is wrong or if we have upset another person. This is why so much context is lost during an email or text message conversation—we can only speculate on their emotional state. It makes sense then that those whom you surround yourself with most often are the people you begin to emulate.

There is a second type of empathy that exists that is referred to as *cognitive empathy*, which involves a more objective experience. It is described as an intellectual understanding of someone else's position, yet the observer does not actually feel the emotions themselves. Cognitive empathy is processed by the temporal-parietal-junction (TPJ) system, and is activated when we are in social situations. Loneliness is known to lead to an atrophy of the TPJ, which explains why it can also lead to the tendency to become socially awkward, further exasperating the situation. Loneliness also decreases the activity of the ventral tegmental area, resulting in lower wellbeing, but our habits are subject to the habits of those we associate ourselves with. We have already learned the power of following our own intuition and the importance of adhering to goals that inspire us, as it relates to dopamine and addiction. When faced with the challenges of wanting to live in accordance with your own truth, and also desiring to feel loved and accepted, it can seem as if you can do only one of two things or, as I would highly recommend, you can do both.

How?

- **Find a network of people with similar ideas and interests**. Surround yourself with those you want to emulate. Attend events and lectures with those who share your vision. Join a gym or fitness class so you can find peers who value the lifestyle you want to adopt. Associate yourself with the kinds of people you want to learn something from, and with whom you can share your ideas.
- **Educate those around you and become a leader**. Share your knowledge and be of service to your existing community by educating them. Be yourself, and have faith that with enough conviction in your actions, those around you will begin to mimic your behaviour. Order the salad when everyone else is having pizza, and be confident in your execution. You never know, maybe someone else at the table also wanted the salad, but was too scared to do so out of fear of being ridiculed. When you walk your path with certainty, you convince others that it's safe to do the same. As a result of your courage the whole community benefits, because the level of awareness expands for the collective group.

I'd like to make the distinction between what I refer to as "service to the community" and altruism. Altruism is sacrificing your resources (time, money, or energy) for no personal gain. Service to a community, by my definition, is providing a service for the betterment of humanity while receiving an equal gain, whether that gain is monetary wealth, social status, spiritual advancement, or whatever else that is valuable to you as an individual. There needs to be some kind of personal profit that you are aware of and you are satisfied with. Without a fair exchange, you risk two things—breeding resentment for those you are serving, or permitting yourself to be the subordinate in society. Why is that important when it comes to the subject of emotional eating? Well, while I am sure there are some instances when subordinating may be thrilling, as a general rule, subservience and empowerment don't mix.

Serotonin (also referred to by some as the "leadership hormone") is involved in the regulation of mood, appetite, sleep, and other cognitive functions, including memory and learning. In humans, serotonin is primarily found in the gastrointestinal tract, and mediates gut movement and perception of resources—including social status and dominance. In response to perceived scarcity, abundance, dominance, or submission, our mood and appetite may be lowered due to this neurotransmitter. As we know already, serotonin is an appetite suppressant, and that is due to its ability to halt dopamine release.

In macaque alpha males (a species of primates), it was found that twice the level of serotonin was released in the brain than in subordinate males. It seemed that social hierarchy and serotonin levels were correlated. Once the dominant males were removed, the other males began to compete for dominance. Males who at one time were subordinate now established dominance, and serotonin levels of the new dominant individuals also increased to double those in subordinate males.

Your life is precious, and your time is a commodity that can never be returned. Expend it wisely among those who not only value you, but also uplift you.

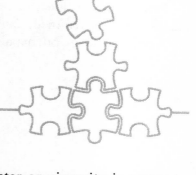

CHAPTER 7

Sincerity

Simply put, this chapter on sincerity is meant to encourage you to be your own authority when it comes to your wellness journey, to allow yourself to think independently despite the onslaught of opposing nutritional information out there ready to be consumed. I'd like to remind you not to fall prey to herd-like mentality by simply permitting yourself to download some of society's most erroneous lines of thinking; just because the vast majority regards something as true, it doesn't actually make it a fact. Be sceptical in your investigations if something doesn't quite sit right with you; question it. Listening to the feedback of your own body is much more vital to your recovery than subscribing to the ideas cast upon us by society.

The phrase "everything in moderation" sends a chill down my spine every single time I hear it. I often (and when I say often, I mean always) respond with "even crystal meth?" At which point, I prepare myself for a lengthy debate on semantics. The most insistent people proclaim that I have taken the words too literally, which reveals to me that there is some arbitrary line when it comes to translating the "everything" in this particular phrase.

Where is the line in this capricious statement? The same level of sanity that assumes it would be absurd to suggest that crystal meth could be taken in moderation should assume that any other substance that is detrimental to our health would apply. Yet, it is considered foolish to include meth, but wise to include other harmful addictive substances, such as refined white sugar, which is laced in so many "foods." When it comes to addictions such as drugs, alcohol, or gambling, we respect the need for the addict to completely abstain. But for those struggling with an addiction to sugar, we devalue one another's decision to renounce it, and we downplay the consequences to our lives if we endorse keeping it in our diet.

There are some foods that can be the trigger that causes the food addict to engage in a vicious downward spiral of uncontrollable binge eating. Some of the most common culprits that lead to this destructive mess are: refined white sugar, high-fructose corn syrup, refined wheat products, sweetened chocolate, refined fat, and excessively salty foods, among a few others. Sugar, for example, mimics the effects of cocaine by sharing the same neuropathways and neurochemicals as cocaine, while it's believed that flour tempers moods and can have a numbing effect on pain, just like an anesthetic. Sweetened chocolate has been studied for its opioid effect that is similar to alcohol. It may also be that chocolate interacts with neurotransmitters such as dopamine (chocolate contains tyrosine, which is the precursor to dopamine), serotonin, and endorphins (contained in

83

chocolate) that contribute to appetite, reward, and mood regulation.

All of these foods, which pose an enormous threat when it comes to binge eating, are manufactured by the food industry and are designed to be highly pleasurable, so much so that we find them euphoric. The food industry has been so effective at engineering these immensely rewarding foods that in some people, simply a tiny taste of a particular trigger food can spark an insatiable appetite that cannot be controlled by the food addict. Trigger foods can vary from person to person; what is innocuous to one person can be an irresistible drug to another. When it comes to trigger foods, complete abstinence from that particular refined or engineered food is crucial.

The expression "I'd rather die happy" gives me an even greater visceral reaction because it implies that unhealthy eating behaviour actually brings you more joy than adopting healthy habits. This fallacy could not be any more antagonistic to the sanctity of your life.

Let's face it; taking responsibility for your health, initially, can feel painful. It requires withdrawal from your favourite foods, time away from relaxing on the couch; it often means you have to learn to pre-plan meals, and perhaps even adopt the habit of carrying a snack-pack full of carrots, just in case hunger strikes at an inopportune time or place. Then, of course, there is that social factor again. It's not uncommon for those around you to so generously provide you with ample opportunities to display that willpower you have been so actively exercising.

Imagine it; you are chomping down on your carrots whilst your coworker has a glazed donut in hand that they are about to inhale, and then you hear it. "Carrots? Are you a rabbit?"

It took a lot of self-reflection to come to a place in life where being called a rabbit for eating salad didn't derail my progress by making me feel a sense of shame. Picture this all too familiar scenario: while stuffing their respective face with that donut, one says, "Well, I'd rather eat this and die happy." A temporary moment of deep panic sets in as you fear you may not have your priorities straight anymore. This statement somehow convinces you that you are going to wither down to the size of a rabbit and may die a miserable, old hag! Oh yeah, "I'd rather die happy..." why didn't I think of that? Well, if eating whatever your heart desires makes you happy, then who can argue with that? Oh, wait... that's right, I can!

What is critical to remember when you are called a rabbit is that unless they are planning on dying in the next few minutes with that donut in their hands, then they will not die any happier than the person who learned to say no to instant gratification. In actuality, if one's goal at the end of their life is to in fact "die happy," then they would need to very carefully step away from the donut and arm themselves with a few new (and healthy) habits instead.

<u>5 Ways to Die Happier</u>

#1. A lifetime of curiosity

It has become common knowledge that overconsumption of sugar is a primary factor in developing type 2 diabetes (insulin resistance). Type 2 diabetes is an extremely debilitating disease that can rob you of many of the joys in life, such as sight and mobility. This disease can ultimately lead to blurred vision, nerve damage, and loss of feeling in your feet. But what many of us aren't aware of is that researchers have believed for some time that there is a strong link between type 2 diabetes and dementia. I don't know about you, but I don't believe you can die happy if you can't remember any of the things in life you are happy about.

The old adage "Use it or lose it" very much applies to your brain. Continually using your brain and learning new things has proven to keep your mind sharp well into your older years. You could even take advantage and double up by educating yourself on what it truly takes to live longer and happier.

Physical exercise is known to stimulate a variety of processes that enhance health and longevity in the brain as well as the body. During aerobic exercise, once your blood starts pumping, a substance likened to Miracle-Gro for the brain, called brain-derived neuro-trophic factor (BDNF), huddles near the synapses. As a result of this activity, more BDNF receptors are stimulated and increased, enhancing our memory due to positive effects on the hippocampus.

#2. Protect your heart

I've previously explained how a high-sugar diet can ultimately lead to increased abdominal fat. Research shows that those with increased abdominal fat are at greater risk of developing heart disease. While I have been fortunate enough to have never had to experience watching someone die of a heart attack, I'd say it's safe to assume that they didn't die smiling. People with excessive belly fat tend to have higher levels of the stress hormones cortisol and adrenaline, which would indicate that not only are they no happier, but they are actually more stressed-out.

The good news is that a whole food, high-fibre diet, rich in essential fatty acids, is associated with a decreased risk of developing heart disease.

#3. Be all in

The nutrients you get from your diet are what your brain needs to make "feel-good hormones" like serotonin or dopamine. Nutrient deficiencies can mean that your brain literally cannot produce the chemicals that evoke good feelings. Even one missing nutrient can pose a threat. It's kind of like baking—you leave one thing out and the whole recipe is a write-off. You may say to me, "Can I eat a salad and then eat the donut?" The truth is... not really. The nutrients you need to digest a particular food are found in the food itself, unless it has been refined. Because refined foods are stripped of their nutrients, they can actually steal from your body the nutrients they need to be metabolized. Many of the nutrients missing in refined sugar—that it then loots from your body—are the exact nutrients your brain would require to make pleasure-inducing chemicals.

You can increase absorption and assimilation of nutrients by working on digestive health. Eliminating refined or processed foods, eating a variety of whole foods, drinking plenty of water between meals, thoroughly chewing your meals, eating only when you are actually hungry (not bored, craving, or overeating), and keeping a peaceful state of mind at mealtimes are some of the most effective ways to support the digestive system. This makes it easier to obtain adequate levels of nutrition for all your body's biochemical processes.

#4. Abort the roller coaster

The reason one might initially feel happy when they eat sugar is largely because sugar causes large amounts of dopamine to be released in your brain. When large quantities are released at once—or all day long, for that matter—the dopamine receptors in your brain then down-regulate. Down-regulated dopamine receptors means your brain needs to release even more of this hormone than it would regularly need to, just to feel normal. The result is you feel depressed; until, of course, you get your next hit. Just like any highly addictive pleasure-inducing substance, over time you need more and more, not only to feel the same high, but simply to feel normal.

Instead, fill your diet with a variety of plant-based foods, such as fruits and vegetables. Over time, you'll find that fruits are all the sweet you need.

#5. Decorate your plate

In order to get up off the couch and want to exercise, you need motivation. How does one feel motivated? Oh yes, that would be dopamine again. Dopamine is the neurotransmitter that regulates motivation. So in other words: no dopamine, no motivation. This is why depressed individuals tend to have little desire to even get out of bed in the morning.

Live, plant-based foods that are vibrant in colour are packed with nutrients, antioxidants, amino acids, and fibre, all of which are especially beneficial to your health. Each colour is unique in the essential nutrients it contains. Neurotransmitters and energy production both rely on a nutritious diet. To help avoid nutritional deficiencies and to ensure a wholesome, balanced diet, it is important to incorporate an abundance of all colours of the rainbow. When preparing each meal, one of my main goals is to decorate my plate with a prism of colours—greens, blue, yellow, red, orange, purple, and so on. Of course, not every plate needs to contain all the colours, but as a general rule, I aim to consume all these colours in the span of a day. I hope it's obvious when I say that lollies don't count.

So there you have it. When it comes to your health, ignorance is not bliss. I'm no human happiness calculator, but more sickness, less memory, more belly fat, more stress, less motivation and purpose, don't add up to more happiness to me by any means. I believe there is no worse fate than being trapped in a miserable body. If you would agree, then don't be fooled by nonsensical remarks such as, "I'd rather die happy."

The Cheat Day

Who came up with the bright idea of the cheat day, and how did we all get convinced that it's a good idea? A very long time ago, I was one of those people. Six days out of the week you adopt wholesome eating patterns, and then one day a week you eat anything you want, with no regard for your health. Many endorse the cheat day in the same way they have accepted the idea of "everything in moderation." The cheat day philosophy allows us to excuse our gluttonous behaviour, and it insinuates that somehow on the seventh day, your body is immune to the ill effects of binging—which simply isn't true. As crazy as it may sound, your digestive system, immune system, and all the other bodily systems work exactly the same way, no matter what day of the week it happens to be. What is detrimental to your health on Monday is equally unfavourable on Saturday.

What I find most offensive about this scheme is its capacity to restrict us from ever really breaking free. It generally takes about 21 to 30 days to make or break a habit, depending on the individual. But it's more like 90 days before the new habit becomes second nature (a key indicator of why "The Eating Enigma" program is a protocol that must be followed for 90 days). Unfortunately, the 21 to 30 days it takes to begin to adopt a new habit need to be consecutive days. If one makes wise nutritional decisions for six consecutive days, and then takes a break on the seventh day, then what would have been their eighth day is now the first day, and they would need at least 20 more days to effectively change the habit. Having a cheat day once every week means you never really become unchained. This pattern only cheats us from ever making a long-term change.

Besides the limitations this concept sets on your habits, it inhibits the likelihood that you will enjoy the taste of a more wholesome meal plan in the future. Almost all of us factor in how palatable food will be when we make our food decisions. Based on our previous experience, our taste buds help cast the vote on determining if we feel like eating it. We know that our taste buds become desensitized over time. We eventually need more chili on our plate, or an extra teaspoon of sugar in our coffee, or extra salt on our chips. Suddenly, fruit is not sweet enough, despite the inherent nutrient density, and it takes second place to dessert. Sure, it takes some time with a healthier meal plan before you actually enjoy it, but it doesn't take as long as most believe it does for us to go back to our natural sense of taste. The average life of a taste bud is only 10 days. Regrettably, a cheat day every seventh day drastically decreases the likelihood you will truly enjoy what you're eating the other six days. The longer you go without cheating with processed foods, the more delectable nature will start to taste.

Choosing the Right Nutritional Advice

What if your local grocer had a sign on display that read, "Purchase your overpriced heroin here."

Not sold?

How about if they very cleverly package it with the word "Organic" on it? Or "Vegan," "Gluten-free," "Reduces appetite," or, "No sugar added"? Oh, I know: "Fat-free!"

We are taught from a young age that heroin, no matter where you buy it, how much it costs, or how cleverly it is packaged, is garbage. When it comes to what we eat, we have a harder time distinguishing between what is healthy and what is trash.

91

As a general rule, if we'd be extremely concerned if our dogs got into it and ate it, then we should probably be worried just the same as if we eat it. All jokes aside, thanks to brilliant marketing, it is becoming increasingly harder to know how to properly read a food label, and then to accurately assess if it's nutritious or toxic.

For the most part, real food is not preserved in a package, which eliminates the space to write these tricky little labels or a list of ingredients. Real foods (healthy foods) have a short shelf life, are one ingredient long, can't be stored in a cardboard box in your pantry for months, and are unrefined whole foods. So, if you are reading a label, then that is a good sign it's not going to qualify as a healthy food option.

With that said, in this day and age, packaged foods are so popular for a reason; they are convenient, and they aren't going anywhere anytime soon. When buying these foods you can read the labels, and do your best to determine which of the options is better for your body. Words like "natural" or "calories" should have little to do with your decision. To me, it's all about the quality and quantity of the actual ingredients. Let me help make reading these labels a little less deceiving.

Labels

Each food in its natural, unrefined state contains all the nutrients needed for your body to properly metabolize it. For example, raw sugar cane, before being separated into two parts—refined white sugar and blackstrap molasses—can actually be considered healthy because it contains some nutrients. Our body recognizes it, can metabolize it, and can readily obtain nutrients from it. (Still, large quantities of excessively sweet foods would negatively impact your body due to other factors, such as hyperglycaemia.) White sugar is devoid of its nutrients, so in order to digest it, it must steal from your body all the vitamins, minerals, and amino acids required to metabolize it. Furthermore, refined sugar is robbed of its fibre. Fibre is good for many reasons, but one is that it slows down the rate at which a food is digested. This is important because it reduces the rate at which the sugar will be released into your bloodstream, decreasing the likelihood of a rapid spike in blood sugar and insulin (the fat-storing hormone).

Carbohydrates that break down rapidly during digestion have a higher glycemic index. High-GI foods release their glucose into the blood quickly, causing a spike to our blood glucose levels. Refined and processed sweeteners are among the top of the list. Studies show that chronic consumption of high-GI foods may lead to chronically high oxidative stress, which has been shown to damage fatty acids. Fatty acids are essential to the composition of the brain, so oxidative damage from a high-GI diet is correlated to dulling of the brain.

Ingesting excessive sugar and other refined junk food can impair one's ability to think clearly and maintain balanced emotions. For these reasons, among many others, it's best to ditch products with added sweeteners. Of course, I do understand that it's not always easy to go cold turkey. My top three choices for added sweeteners are dates, honey, and maple syrup, simply because consuming these doesn't mean the body has to be pillaged of its own nutrients in order to digest it. But, there is something more to consider. Even some natural sweeteners can be trigger foods due to their excessively sweet taste or their high levels of fructose. Fructose, in excessive amounts, can interfere with leptin. If you remember from an earlier chapter, leptin is the satiating hormone that signals us to put down our forks. Foods like high-fructose corn syrup and other processed foods can be trigger foods because of their contribution to leptin resistance.

There's also the "5 ingredients or less" rule. The rule is, don't buy anything that contains more than five ingredients. Again, five ingredients or less doesn't necessarily classify it as wholesome, but I do think it's a good idea to avoid most products that have more than five ingredients in them. The greater number of ingredients can (and usually does) mean more processing, leading to a greater toxic load. This is especially true if it sounds like one or more of those ingredients were made in a laboratory.

One of the following just doesn't belong here. Can you guess what it is?

- Apple
- Almond
- Artificial sweetener

Start by giving yourself more credit. We can all identify the difference between what Mother Nature provides us and what was made in a factory, and that distinction is all we really need. Go with your gut, not a fancy label. While it's true that when buying produce, organic is often a better choice, that doesn't apply to everything in a package. Don't be a sucker for marketing, fancy brown paper bags, or expensive price tags. A creative campaign never trumps the extraordinary intelligence of Mother Nature.

Counting Calories

Although initially effective for some at controlling weight, counting calories, in my opinion, is not a sustainable nor healthy way of managing weight. Over the long-term, it can increase anxiety around mealtime, and can lead to poor dietary decisions. A large avocado can contain as many as 400 calories, but a chocolate bar can contain approximately half of that amount. Counting calories as a means of dietary management suggests that it is better to eat the chocolate bar over the avocado that is loaded with nutrition. An avocado contributes nearly 20 vitamins, minerals, and beneficial plant compounds, as well as healthy monounsaturated fats and beneficial soluble fibre to our bodies. Meanwhile, a chocolate bar may take you temporarily into a state of bliss, but it will do nothing for you on the nutritional level; they are incomparable.

In addition, attempting to restrict calories by means of food deprivation is associated with binge eating. Laboratory rats deprived of food for as little as two hours consumed significantly more calories during their next opportunity to eat than rats that were not deprived.

Eating Superfoods

For a nutritionist, the word *superfood* is kind of a double-edged sword. I am excited about this trend, and encourage people to eat superfoods. I can only hope my new term "superfood me" one day grows to be as well-known as "supersize me." On the flip side, I fear that following this trend without educating oneself can actually lead to nutritional deficiencies, allergies, and binge eating by focusing on only one popular health food at a time. That said, I understand that not everyone has the time or ability to learn about current nutritional thinking and stay consistently current, but the truth is, not much research is required when identifying super-foods. By definition, a superfood is a nutrient-rich food considered to be especially beneficial to health and wellbeing. It is as simple as that.

An assortment of superfoods does help support a healthy body, but celebrating only one food at a time the way the media has done overlooks the critical importance of a well-balanced diet. As I mentioned earlier, an effortless way of ensuring that your diet is rich in nutrients is by adding the full spectrum of colour from live, plant-based foods into your meal plan. The more chromatic your plate is, the more superfoods it contains, and the more bountiful in essential nutrients it is.

Fruits and vegetables are vibrant in colour, high in nutrients, loaded with beneficial fibre, and relatively low in calories. If your plate is mainly white, beige, or brown, then it's likely lacking a medley of nutrients. Be careful with restricted diets that vilify some of nature's finest foods, like fruits, vegetables, nuts, and seeds, and glorify refined or processed ingredients. Know the distinction between real food and engineered, food-like substances, which in my opinion shouldn't be classified as food at all.

Among real food, there is no one specific food that is coming to kill you, and there is no one specific food that is coming to save you. Eat a variety, and load your diet with as many wholesome, plant-based foods as you can find that are local, in season, and unprocessed.

Ask yourself, "How will I feel after I eat this?" Be authentic to yourself; if you feel sick after you eat it, or it triggers an uncontrollable desire to compulsively eat until you feel sick, then it doesn't matter what anyone else believes about it—you shouldn't eat it! A food addiction works the same as any other substance addiction. Eating one of your trigger foods—even just one bite—can cause you to fall off the wagon and take you back to square one. For a food addict, complete and total abstinence from trigger foods for their entire life is necessary.

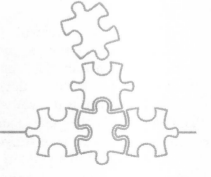

CHAPTER 8

Perception

Our perceptions are strictly bound by the gross limitations of our senses. The human eye can only pick up wavelengths within the limits of about 390 to 700nm. Our ears, tactile senses, and even our taste buds are also all confined to a tiny portion of the potential waveforms that surround us.

We depend on our eyes as the main source of gathering information around us, but our eyes are merely trained to see light and reflected light. In other words, we can only see portions of objects that reflect or emit light confined to a narrow spectrum. Wavelengths outside the human visual spectrum cannot be converted into impulses from the eyes, and thus are not interpreted by the brain. In actuality, the eyes, brain, and mind don't "see" anything. They simply work in unison to translate waveforms. What is ultimately witnessed is subject to the interpretation of the observer.

We don't see much of what is in our visual range if we don't recognize or expect it to be there. We filter out a great deal of what we don't recognize and expect, and much is simply ignored by the mind. This is a magnificent gift that Mother Nature has bestowed upon us; we have the ability to draw in whatever resources we need at that time from our environment. This skill increases our likelihood of obtaining each of our goals, thus ensuring a greater chance of survival. It also means that throughout our entire lives, we are drawing our conclusions from a very tiny percent of the big picture. The remaining truth, we are totally and completely blind to.

Our attention gets the authority to determine what our eyes select to draw in and what doesn't make the cut. Consequently, our attention and focus is governed by our emotions. Our emotions not only spotlight our attention, but they also stimulate our thoughts, beliefs, and behaviours. This perpetuates a feedback cycle each and every time we encounter something. What is important to remember is that two things contribute to maintaining and strengthening our neural networks— repetition and elevated emotion.

No two human brains are exactly alike because none of us share in all the same experiences. Initially, our neurons are organized similarly, but the trillions of new connections are formed over our lifetime, creating vast varieties of neural networks. From before we are born to the moment we take our last breath, the brain undergoes extensive cellular change. These intricate little networks that are formed from life experiences differ quite drastically from person to person. What each of us sees on the outside is very much a projection of what we feel on the inside. If you came into this world with the same brain and body, but had a completely different history— and thus altered emotional states—your perceptions of both the world and yourself would be transformed significantly as a reflection of that history.

The brain collects the small percentage of data our eyes pick up, draws its interpretations from it, organises it, and uses the information to build on what it has already learned in the past. I say that it draws its interpretations because that's exactly what they are... interpretations. Even when you believe you saw something, it's not necessarily what was genuinely there.

Have you ever seen two black spots floating around through your vision? That's a truer picture of what you should be seeing. There is a completely blind region in the eye, known as the optical disc. This is where retinal neurons huddle together to make their way into the depths of the brain tissue. The optic disc, which is present in both our eyes, contains no cells that can perceive sight, yet we don't always see these black spots. That is because your brain is a resourceful little magician that picks up the signal from your visual cortex, and then it audits what's 360 degrees around the disc and makes its assumptions through a process called "filling in." Yes, that's right, it just fills in with whatever it believes is most likely to be there, but not necessarily what's veritably there.

What you see at any given moment is your mind's distorted version of reality.

Unless, of course, you're in the midst of learning something completely new, in which case you're required to pay attention to new information; your brain is just filtering the world in through a small funnel that discards material it doesn't deem to be important. In other words, if you have no prior experience with it, you often don't even notice it. Just because something has yet to be granted access through the gates of your eyes by your attention, doesn't also mean it doesn't exist.

Moreover, societal pressures seem to play a huge role in how we interpret sensory information. If family members, friends, or research make suggestions to us, it has the ability to distort our perceptions. Our observations seem to be highly prone to suggestibility.

The Asch conformity experiments were a series of studies conducted by social psychologist Solomon Asch of Swarthmore College that were published in the 1950s. The study demonstrated the potential influence of conformity within groups. In the experiment, students were asked to participate in a group vision test. Each person in each group was asked questions, and had to provide answers about a length of a line they observed. In reality, all but one of the participants was asked to answer the question incorrectly. To avoid the "real" participant from having a sense of what was actually going on, the other participants gave the obvious, correct answer on the first two trials. On the third trial, however, the other participants then gave the wrong answer. The purpose of the study was to see if the remaining student would react differently based on the other subjects' answers. When the wrong answer was provided by the group, the "real" subjects often also responded incorrectly. This was opposed to the control group, with no pressure to conform, where only 1 participant out of 35 answered incorrectly.

Over time, we establish beliefs about people and circumstances, and we have this innate knack to draw in from the world that which supports our beliefs. We look for evidence to confirm how we already feel. Rarely do we seek proof to negate what we have already decided to be true.

For example, let's say that I offered you a pill — we can call it pill X — and I told you that if you took it, you would grow taller. If you wanted to believe that, you would type into your search engine "pill x and getting taller." As a direct result of the words you typed, you would likely find some sort of assurance to buy into the pill. If you didn't believe that a pill could make you taller, or perhaps you lacked trust in me, you would be more inclined to type "pill x and myths about getting taller" into your search engine, at which point you may find drastically different content, strengthening your case against my claims.

Another example is how we feel about people in general. If we label people as inherently bad, we pay more attention to the different ways we can be at risk. When we see or hear news about someone doing something bad, we have a strong emotional reaction. The deep emotion it evokes makes it more likely that we store and remember it. The truth really is that people are just people, and they do both kind things and cruel things. Had you looked with unbiased eyes, you would have seen evidence of both. This rule also applies to the way you see yourself.

Here's what I am getting at; if you have never seen your own magnificence, felt inner love and contentment, or been able to imagine anything greater for your life than what you already know, it doesn't mean it's not well and truly out there completely within your reach. The emotions you feel are filtering your reality and confirming what you already believe. Your attention has exclusive command over the admissions of your gate. Lucky for you, should you choose, you can use your consciousness to direct your awareness.

It's not just your current perception of reality that is skewed either. Your ability to accurately reflect on the events of your past, or to see the potential possibilities in your future, is heavily influenced by the limitations of your current state of mind.

There is a term known as *delayed discounting*, which is our inclination to value an immediate gain over a long-term reward—even if the long-term benefits actually have the same or greater value. Not only do we overly appraise immediate rewards, but we also discount the delayed risks or consequences as well.

Let's say I told you that in one year's time I would give you $500, but if you waited just one additional month, then I would give you $550. Would you wait the extra month? If you are anything like most people, you would opt to take the 10 percent interest and wait that extra month—it's a no-brainer. What if I told you I would give you $500 today or you could wait a month and I would give you $550; does that change your answer?

In the second scenario, most people would prefer to choose the instant gratification over long-term gain. Both of these scenarios require you to wait for the same length of time to get the same 10 percent return, but scenario #2 offers another variable that scenario #1 doesn't offer, and that is known as "now appeal."

Now appeal is a term used to describe the tendency we have to allow our current emotional state to be factored into the equation while being partial to that emotional state by letting it bear more weight than the quantitative future risks or rewards. Yet another shining example of how our perceptions in the present may alter our visions of the future. Moreover, our emotions in our present life are subject to the perception of the past. So you can see how we let our past determine our future.

Now that I have spent all of this time coercing you into the idea of opening your mind to a brand-new future, we may want to go back and revisit our old friend surrogacy again.

There is a famous marshmallow study on delayed discounting that took place in the late 1960s and early 1970s led by psychologist Walther Mischel, who was a professor at Stanford University. In these studies, a child was offered a choice between one small reward (a marshmallow, cookie, or pretzel) which they could have immediately, or double that reward if they waited for a short period of approximately 15 minutes. The researchers found that the children who waited for the long-term rewards kept their minds distracted by doing other things. Ah yes, we covered this gem of a trick in the chapter on surrogacy.

I've already discussed the importance of allowing yourself to have a greater goal that conflicts with the desire to compulsively eat. From where you're currently standing, that greater goal may only appear to be obtainable in the distant future. That perspective alone puts your greater goal at risk to the biased eyes of now appeal. It is equally important to have daily goals and action steps that we can take towards that new future. It is increasingly beneficial to preoccupy oneself during a craving with one of those daily action steps towards the new goal.

Dopamine levels rise with anticipation. Knowing that just beyond the doors of your freezer is a tub of mint chocolate ice cream, but that swimsuit season is still eight months away, will be enough to convince you that starting your new life tomorrow would be a much better idea. As soon as you retrieve the goal (in this case, the ice cream), you can see the errors in your logic, but by then it's too late.

Avoid this fallacy by filling your space with reminders of what you really want. Remove temptations from your space, and keep your eyes on the prize — your wellbeing. Set small targets every day, and make small or large steps toward a life that is truly fulfilling to you. Anticipate new goals and healthy habits that are also just within reach. Cravings are created from a cue in the environment. Responding to that trigger with a new routine trains the brain to adopt a new habit, as long as that new routine ultimately ends with a rewarding feeling.

Our memories of the past grossly impact both our current perception of reality and our future potential, if we allow it to. Most of us permit the information we have already retained to dictate our future, and in many instances, this process can protect us. But it also frames our future potentials as well. In reality, we can't rely on our memories to accurately reflect what we truly have experienced in the past. In this case, we are confined by the limitations of our imperfect memory.

There are a few types of memory, but I'd like to focus on the two most popularly known — short-term memory and long-term memory. When we experience an event, the brain doesn't just gather the information and store it in one place. Rather, our senses pick up the data, our brain dissects it, and then the information gets stored in completely different regions within the brain. For example, signals from your sight are routed to the visual cortex and into the occipital lobe.

105

Sounds that are processed through your ears are consequently transported to the auditory cortex. Hundreds of different regions in the brain can be used to store just one memory.

Of course, we don't seem to be able to recall everything we experience. We are far more likely to remember something if it is linked with a strong emotion, or if the memory is interesting or meaningful to us, and we seem to forget a huge majority of the other things we experienced throughout our lifetime. The brain also has a tendency to focus more on the gist of the story, rather than the specifics of the event.

Short-term memory, also known as working memory, is an accumulation of temporary memories. Working memory is the link between the initial moments of processing information and the consolidation of long-term memories. Consolidation is a mechanism that escorts short-term memory into long-term memory. New memories are fragile, easily amendable, and subject to extinction; but if something is considered to be valuable information or emotionally interesting, then it is stored, becoming a long-term memory.

It was believed that once long-term memories were established, they could not return to their original flexible conditions. New findings suggest that previously consolidated memories are reverted to short-term memories again when they are recalled from long-term storage. This process has been coined *reconsolidation*. If consolidation is not fixed to a single event, but rather reoccurs each time we reactivate a memory, then the memories that we never recall are the only truly permanent memories we have. If this is the case, memories that are recalled could fall victim to current emotional states, suggestibility, and bias.

In 1962, Daniel Offer, a psychologist in Chicago, began a long-term study involving a group of teenagers. He interviewed 73 male high school students, asking them various personal questions such as: which child in the family did they believe was their mother's favourite? Were they physically punished as discipline? The interviews covered a broad range of topics, such as hobbies, religion, sexuality, self-image, and various other thoughts and beliefs. In 1997, Offer contacted the participants again, asking them many of the same questions, but they were asked to answer as their younger self. The question 35 years later was now: When you were 13, who did you think was your mother's favourite?

As it turned out, during the first interview, 90 percent of the teenagers answered yes to physical punishment, such as being spanked, but only a third of them recalled this information in 1997. In addition, 15 percent of the young men had answered that they were their mother's favourite in 1962, but that number doubled to 30 percent when they were asked many years later.

Our beliefs about our life and what is meant for us in our future is profoundly affected by heavily filtered, distorted perceptions of our past and present-day situations. Our perceptions of the people, events, and circumstances in our lives are merely personal interpretations that favour our emotional state. Our emotions have the ability to serve as a lens filter, funneling external information and reaffirming limiting beliefs. I like to refer to it as though we wear emotional goggles that only invite more of the same into our mind.

Your attention works as the gatekeeper of your garden. We have the ability to direct it, if we choose, but many of us fail to use it to our full advantage. Because of our good friend dopamine, our desires and, consequently, our goals, have the power to govern our attention. We become focused when we see the prospect of our goals, and then our external environment is filtered through the lens of that goal, making each goal exceedingly easier to obtain. New goals allow you to see new prospects, events, and opportunities that you may have otherwise failed to observe. It's a double-edged sword because we all too often stop ourselves from setting goals that are truly valuable to us, based on the limited beliefs we hold about our life and our personal value to the world.

To open the gates of your mind, you have to be willing to turn the locks by shifting your already established beliefs. Most of which, you can now understand, are compiled of misleading evidence from false perceptions anyhow. Based on the emotional goggles the observer has chosen to wear, the outcome of a given scenario can appear quite different from person to person. That outcome drives our beliefs and further steers our perceptions, which keeps us stuck in our moods, and all this ultimately forms what we call our personality. To make matters worse, and to truly keep ourselves disempowered, we begin to assign labels to ourselves.

Behaviours that are a huge detriment to our personal wellbeing are allowed to repeat themselves simply because of assumptions we make about who we are. "I am this way because of my parents," "I am an anxious person," "I am not good at math," "I am not good at sport," "I am impulsive," "I am unlucky," "I am optimistic," "I am lazy," "I am sarcastic," "I am an introvert;" these are nothing but labels that we assign to ourselves. We excuse our behaviour to fit in accordance with these false ideas. Our behaviour then reaffirms the belief, and we deem it as some sort of evidence. If we excuse the behaviour on several occasions, we then regard it as a fact about ourselves, then name it to be one of the characteristics of our personality.

We have all had a change of mind and heart before. What happens in these instances? Typically, something meaningful has caused us to change our perception of a person, place, or event.

Where we stand on a matter is dependent on where we currently sit. If you believe you are not destined for a particular goal, then data reaffirming that opinion finds its way into your secret garden and is stored in the recesses of your mind. That data is consequently trans-lated into thoughts and carried forth in habits, actions, and behaviours. But the opposite is also true; if you open your mind, begin to believe in your vast poten-tial, and allow yourself to witness this evidence, you filter into your garden only that which supports those empowering beliefs. Any data that doesn't support that belief is disregarded, as it is not pertinent information in regards to the direction that you have chosen to head.

In order to obtain new goals, we have to dissipate limiting beliefs so we can set new intentions that are governed by altered emotional states. As soon as our actions and behaviours start to match our inner inten-tions, we begin to embody the person we truly desire to be. Once the mind and body are working in harmony towards a goal, the observer's personal reality begins to reflect the new personality.

In conjunction, the words "I am" are the two most powerful weapons we can use to either work against us, or in favour of us. So please use them wisely when you envision your ideal life.

We live in a time when we are obsessed with cause and effect. Being visual animals, we tend to want to witness our greatness before we can believe it's true. Unfortunately, in order to witness something, we need to expect that it already exists. To birth a change that has yet to materialise in the present reality, the creator has to hold faith. Otherwise, no advancement can be made and we become stuck, creating more of what we already know—which isn't really creation at all, now is it? Nothing demonstrates the power of our beliefs quite like the placebo effect.

The phenomenon commonly called the placebo effect or placebo response is when a person who is given an ineffectual treatment, such as a sugar pill, sham surgery, or other various treatment, has a perceived or actual improvement in their condition. Brain imaging techniques have been done showing that a placebo can have real, measurable effects on physiological changes in the brain. In the opposite effect, nocebo is when a person who disbelieves in a treatment experiences a worsening of their symptoms or listed possible side effects, even though they have been provided the ineffectual treatment, such as the sugar pill.

The placebo effect and self-fulfilling prophecies are one and the same. Both are predictions that cause themselves to come true due to feedback between belief, physiology, and behaviours.

It's not uncommon for people to set their limitations based on their perceptions, but to blame their inactions on their imagination. "I could never imagine myself doing that," they might say. In actuality, what their mind has just done is imagined it, compared it to what they already know, calculated their personal value based on what they have experienced in the past. They then determined if the vision was possible for them. Imagination then, is not to blame. You can imagine yourself doing anything. You can imagine yourself riding a unicorn on a moon in a distant galaxy if you want to, but just because you can envision something, doesn't also mean you believe in it. Therefore, it is your beliefs—the ones you accumulated from your perceptions of past and present experiences—that block the flow of expressing your imagination.

I have provided you with logical insight into how our perception of the world is simply a projection of what's inside our own mind. The intention here is to now invite you to abandon the fictitious perceptions and beliefs about the person you think you are. Instead, embody the person you want to be so you can fill your mind and heart with love and admiration for yourself and your life. A fulfilled heart leads to a purposeful life, and thus fills the void that we are tempted to stuff with food and various stimulants.

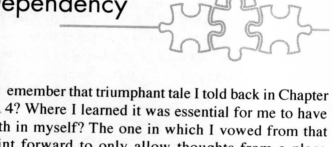

CHAPTER 9

Dependency

Remember that triumphant tale I told back in Chapter 4? Where I learned it was essential for me to have faith in myself? The one in which I vowed from that point forward to only allow thoughts from a place of love for myself to live, grow, and flourish inside of my mind?

It's a good story... if I didn't eventually revert back to my old way of being.

Sometimes we have the best intentions to change but it seems within mere days, weeks, or sometimes months, we fall off course. Well, sure, we know will-power has something to do with that, but what about our emotional state? In a moment when you make a pledge to yourself that you are going to change, you are typically in an overly elevated emotional state. So either you're feeling exceptionally down and never want to feel that way again, so you vow to change, or you're elated and you want to continue to feel that way. Either way, you're not being your typical self. On an average day where nothing really significant happens, we don't feel a spark to make drastic alterations to our lives. When someone reaches rock bottom, the emotion can be so powerful that it often does make some kind of difference long-term. Although in my case I was not at rock bottom, so it didn't impact me to the same degree.

I had come to a realization that sparked a light inside me, but eventually that light just faded away. I did plant new, loving thoughts in my mind, but the old ones were still there and they stole the cake.

I was never going to become someone else with new habits, and my life would never be any different if old emotions that governed my actions were still dominating my life. We can learn an endless stream of life lessons and we can convince ourselves that we get the point, but until we simultaneously prune out old thinking, we will continue to live in the same rut of trying and failing. This is because, in this case, the body has been conditioned to control the mind. In order to have long-term success, we have to recondition the mind along with the body.

Think of your thoughts as the vocabulary of your mind and your emotions as the vocabulary of your body. Each thought we have evokes a corresponding emotion, which we get to experience through our feelings. While some of these thoughts provoke us to feel a substantial physiologic shift, some others are much less significant, generating a more delicate response within the body. All of our thoughts have one thing in common—they all have the power to send specific instructions to the body on how it should respond. Chemical messengers travel through the nervous system, and they spark a physiological change in less than a second. In a sincerely troublesome situation where our lives are at risk, this rapid reaction time could mean the difference between life and death.

For instance, imagine you're driving in your car on your regular route to work; you may be daydreaming about work or listening to an audiobook. All of a sudden, the car in front of you slams on their brakes. Immediately you're alert, and you either slam on your brakes or swerve into the other lane. You were quickly prepared for the peril ahead by the hormones of stress. That nearly instantaneous communication between the mind and the body is what saved the day. Some trouble arises, however, when we are actually safe but we can't turn the stress response off.

If we lived only in the now, and we focused solely on the present, we would only have thoughts that are pertinent in that immediate space. For most day-to-day scenarios, we aren't in any grave danger, so we would ideally be able to sustain a fairly balanced physiology. For those rare instances when our lives are in jeopardy, we can trust that our awareness will hone in on the threat. The stress response switches on and then our loyal servant—the body—swiftly prepares itself for either fight or flight. It's an enchanting dance that unifies the two. The mind leads, and the body willfully follows. It's of service to us, and if it's played out when there is a real threat present, the stress response is our friend.

If we genuinely did live in the moment, we'd be attuned to the fact that we are fairly safe most of the time. We typically wouldn't need to be in that amped-up state. Unless we were in immediate danger, the emotions we feel throughout the body should ideally be ones of peaceful reflection of that present moment. However, a more common practice is to be either obsessing about a past event that we can never change or worrying about some imagined possible future outcome that we are convinced will actually happen. In reality, if you considered all the potential future outcomes, statistically speaking, that future imagined scenario is highly unlikely to occur. Due to creative memory, any past events we are obsessing about might be partly fabricated anyway. Essentially, we spend a lot of our time fantasizing.

That feeling of anxiety about the future is actually the fear of reliving something we've already faced in the past. In other words, there was some moment in the past when we perceived our very survival to be at great risk. We develop an apprehension of re-experiencing that event, or anything that seems remotely similar to it, in our future. When we become consumed by either creative memories and feelings of the past or beliefs and imagined scenarios about the future, we get stuck feeling a specific emotion—often the same one we felt during the original event. Our thoughts alone can spark emotion, and emotion sets the body in motion. Real or imagined, our body can't differentiate between the two.

I think it's fair to assume that we've all faced or will face some significant event that drastically changed the trajectory of our lives, or notably morphed us into a new state of being. Typically, the experience was perceived by the observer to be a tragedy or great loss of some kind. The drastic negative perception during the event evokes a surge of emotion, which then activates the stress response. Once the fight-or-flight response is activated, our senses become extremely acute; the feedback from all of our sensory organs sends information to the brain and jungles of neurons begin to connect, forming a robust memory of that event. The amplitude of the emotion in that time and space is the clincher that really brands us by the event.

In terms of our survival, this snapshot our brain takes in a moment of crisis helps us learn from that experience. That way, we can be better equipped to handle the same crisis the next time around. If, by chance, we re-encounter the same emergency in the future, our mind makes calculations based on both our past training and the new data from the current environment. With that compiled information, it determines the best way to react at that time. When we are confronted with the same challenge on several occasions, we learn from it each time and we become faster, stronger, and wiser (given the threat doesn't kill us). Essentially, each time we are met with the same obstacle, our brains evolve to be better equipped the next time around. It does this by compounding the information that comes from our senses during each encounter with the obstacle. More neurons begin to connect, and the connections begin to wire together stronger in the brain.

Now, if we are forced to face a given stressor regularly, our body starts to make adjustments in response to the redundancy of that stressor, and we become conditioned for an experience. For example, our muscles can get stronger if we exercise physically, or our cardiovascular system adapts if we regularly run, etc.

The same thing occurs in the brain. When you replay a memory, or you repeat a belief about your past experience with enough redundancy while simultaneously rehearsing a specific behaviour to accompany that thought or memory, you condition the body to act in the same pattern every time something triggers that original memory, thought, or belief. So, the thought alone can generate emotion; emotion sends instructions to the body, and the body acts in accordance with previous experience with that emotion. Obsessively thinking about something that actually isn't happening anymore, or has yet to present itself, recreates the experience within the body through thought alone.

The habits we develop are simply by-products of basic conditioning. Negative emotions can feel very uncomfortable, so in order to avoid them, we tend to remedy them with something outside of ourselves to make us feel better. We reach for something pleasurable (in this case, food) to stimulate our senses. This momentarily draws our attention away from the internal displeasure. It works at first, especially when the substance is new to us, because it's known that novel things typically cause us to pay more attention. Not only are we briefly distracted by something we find quite gratifying, but we are also sending ample amounts of new sensory information back to the brain, ensuring that we build on the old experience. Our brain records this new information by forming new circuitry, linking the new data to the old circuits, and ties it to that negative feeling. Over time, our tolerance for the substance (food) inevitably rises, so we need more to silence the storm the next time around. If we self-soothe with food on several occasions, the brain takes that information into consideration and it develops a habit.

Suddenly, food and grief, food and unworthiness, or food and guilt, come in an indivisible pair. The neurons related to the emotion, and the neurons correlated with the substance that gives you a temporary relief from that specific emotion, begin to wire together in the brain. We know that nerve cells that wire together, fire together.

In essence, if one neuron is triggered, the entire jungle lights up simultaneously. Then voila, when you feel that specific emotion, you instantly feel the urgency to eat.

One day, I was working on an extremely enjoyable project. I was in good spirits and all seemed well. Then I realized that every time I got up from that project and I walked into my kitchen to pour myself a glass of water, my thoughts would just instantly shift and I started to worry about all sorts of random things. My brain had literally linked the kitchen and the emotion of worry together. Initially, it was more likely that worrying thoughts would lead me to seek the kitchen. But over time, because neurons that fire together wire together, my brain learned to link the kitchen with nervousness, and eventually, through the magic of neuroplasticity they sang in unison, no matter which of the two had come first.

This insight alone wouldn't have contributed at all to my recovery if I hadn't consciously made the decision to form a new habit. I thought to myself, *If being in the kitchen fires off neurons that are also linked to worrisome feelings and thoughts, and that link formed over time simply because of two things—repetition and elevated emotion—then by that logic, with enough repetition and positive elevated emotion, I should eventually be able to walk into a kitchen and it should subconsciously trigger the new elevated emotion.*

Once I became aware of the link, I could use my awareness while I was in the kitchen to direct my thoughts and I could reprogram my brain. Instead of letting myself fall back into default mode, I made the choice every single time I walked by a kitchen to use my attention to direct my focus to the same positive

118

thought—each and every time. Eventually, and with much rehearsal, new routes did begin to form, and those old networks were subject to extinction.

I remember the day when I realized the new conscious program had become a new subconscious program, as I hadn't even reached the kitchen and already I felt the elevated state. I was in awe that with enough patience and dedication, the mind could convince the body to forget what it once learned.

This is why the activity in Chapter 1 was so important. When we identify our triggers, it gives us some insight. Insight alone really doesn't do anything for us; in fact, in some instances, it can make things worse. Should you choose to marry insight and action, however . . . that is a powerful pair.

When a cue causes us to perform a routine time and time again, it becomes what we would call a habit, or a *nondeclarative memory* (also known as *implicit memory*). Nondeclarative memory is a type of long-term memory that is unlike declarative memory in that it does not require conscious thought. *Procedural memory* is a form of nondeclarative memory that enables us to carry out our most commonly learned tasks without consciously thinking about them; in essence, we can operate on autopilot for many mundane tasks. This frees up our conscious mind so it can be ready to pay attention to and learn new things while we are performing old routine tasks. Riding a bike, walking, tying a shoelace, or brushing our teeth are all exercises we don't need to think much about in order to execute them. We can carry forth these tasks fairly effortlessly, but it's often hard to verbalize exactly how we do them.

In the instance of a food addiction, the action that one plays out perpetually is comfort eating. Emotional eating then gets stored as a nondeclarative memory, as a remedy for a specific emotion and a collection of alternative payoffs. Because they are both wired together in the brain, the behavioural pattern can perpetuate more of the same emotion that one was initially trying to suppress in the first place. The body has associated eating with a specific emotion, and the two not only accompany each other simultaneously, but they now antagonise each other as well. Suddenly, you're stuck in a circuit of thinking, feeling, eating, then more of the same thinking, feeling, and eating.

A single neuron has the potential to establish and maintain connections with about 10,000 other neurons, and each of those neurons can link up to approximately 10,000 other neurons. Essentially, igniting one neuron among the maze has the capacity to kindle an entire labyrinth. This subconscious program of thinking, feeling, and repeating past behaviours becomes devoid of conscious instruction.

According to Dr. Bruce Lipton's book *The Biology of Belief*, it is thought that the subconscious mind processes about 20 million bits of information per second, unlike the conscious mind, which can only process about 40 bits of info per second. Furthermore, the subconscious only operates in the present moment. While our conscious mind may be off in reverie about past and future events and completely oblivious to the majority of the data our subconscious is processing, the subconscious is efficiently regulating our behaviours in any given moment. Now you can appreciate how impulsive behaviour actually works and why the conscious mind could easily miss what the subconscious is up to.

When we become consumed by a belief about our lives, we risk becoming addicted to the emotion associated with it. At the root of any substance dependency can actually be an emotional dependency. This emotional habit is like a subconscious program that has been downloaded from thoughts, and then the routine is memorized by the body. The addiction is not actually the substance itself, as all substances are equally at risk of being abused; we just happened to make the decision to prescribe ourselves food. Rather, the actual addiction is a long-term dependency on the emotional state. Breaking the habit to reach for food doesn't stop the disposition to feel the negative emotion, so eventually, we will find ourselves reaching for something else, transforming our obsessions to some other substance.

In 2012, a ground-breaking study published in the *Journal of the American Medical Association* reported that the percentage of patients abusing alcohol increased significantly in the second year following gastric bypass surgery. Many of these patients insisted that they had no prior problems with drinking before the surgery. Since then, a growing body of evidence has supported these findings. This research could suggest that people might adopt new addictions after weight-loss surgery because they can no longer turn to over-eating as a source of comfort.

The crowning achievement of Mother Earth is adaptability. Throughout time and space, she is flexible to subtle changes and allows for adjustments to her already miraculous design. Each species—from plants to animals—are perfectly primed for their immediate environment. It is this very adaptability that has protected us from going extinct. Adaptation is our super-power. As our environment changes so do we, because our cells respond to the long-term environmental shifts.

When you regularly ruminate over a particular circumstance, you are sending the same signals to the body over a long period of time. As a result of that redundancy, the body believes it has found itself in a new habit. Even though you are no longer physically in the environment where you originally perceived the trauma, reflecting on the emotional event creates changes to the internal physiology. Since the body cannot make the distinction between a real or imagined threat, it makes its necessary adjustments to survive in the new dwelling. We are not designed to be in the stress response for an extended period of time; thus, the body learns to adapt by altering our baseline state. Our external habits (words and actions) are merely a visual manifestation of the internal habitat (thoughts, beliefs, and emotions).

The default baseline of a particular mood is referred to as the *emotional set point*.

Set point theory is supported by research, where it was shown that people who win the lottery, after the initial euphoria has dissipated, are no happier than they were before they won the lottery.

All is not lost though. Up until recently, it was believed that by the time we hit the age of 35, our identity would be completely formed. It was thought that the networks in the brain became hardwired, and thus we ourselves couldn't change, bringing meaning to the phrase, "You can't teach an old dog new tricks." What we now know is that even though some of our circuitry is hardwired (breathing, heartbeat, etc.), our experience-dependent wiring (habits, attitude, beliefs, conditioned responses, skills, etc.) is actually more comparable to software. Learning a new skill, such as a language or a sport, changes your synapses. These connections are therefore more like plastic. It is possible to make the decision to work on your own identity, just as you can make the decision to acquire a new skill. With commitment and persistence, we are able to make new circuits while pruning the old ones, eventually forming a new personality. We can indeed choose to change our state of being.

As we age, our brain's eagerness to evolve is heavily dependent on a number of factors, including adequate nutrients and the substance known as brain-derived neurotrophic factor (BDNF), which can be positively influenced by aerobic exercise. So, our lifestyle choices really do matter.

Richard Davidson, director of the Laboratory for Affective Neuroscience at the University of Wisconsin, discovered that people with a generally more positive disposition had an increased activity level in the left prefrontal cortex (L-PFC). Those who tend to lean more towards depressed or anxious states had heightened activity in the right prefrontal cortex (R-PFC). The amygdala, the part of your brain that operates your emotions, was also kindled along with the R-PFC. In addition, overactivity of the amygdala can be inhibited by the L-PFC.

Rumination is associated with the R-PFC, while practicing focus in the present moment is attributed to the L-PFC. Through continual practice of mindfulness, we are able to alter our emotional set point, because we are increasing activity in the L-PFC. Over time, with enough rehearsal, we find it easier to stay focused, increasing activity in the L-PFC, while decreasing activity of both the amygdala and R-PFC. Details about the amygdala and addiction are beyond the scope of this book, but can be found in the brilliant publication *The Biology of Desire* by Marc Lewis.

Many love to argue that they are "this way" because of their genes. While our genetics do play a significant role, I would like to remind you that our genes have the ability to be expressed in thousands of different ways. The study of epigenetics (above genetics) tells us that our genes are as mutable as our brains.

There are an estimated 100 different neurotransmitters and neurochemicals within the brain. These various messengers work to send signals that cause our cells to express themselves in a variety of ways. The body can be described as a protein-producing factory, as our cells produce proteins. Stomach cells produce enzymes, skin cells produce collagen and elastin, and so on. We express our genes through various cells that produce certain proteins. We also have what are known as "behaviour-state-dependant genes" (activated by stress, emotion, and dreaming) and "experience-dependent genes" (influenced by learning, growth and repair). For the purpose of staying on track, however, I will direct you to *Breaking the Habit of Being Yourself,* by Dr. Joe Dispenza, for more information on these truly fascinating discoveries.

There are a variety of other factors that have the ability to influence our mood and temperament, with the most common culprits being: poor diet, blood sugar imbalance, sleep deprivation, and lack of physical exercise. With repeated insult, each has the ability to affect our state of being.

The heartbreaking reality is this: emotional eating binges and spells of starving oneself are often two sides of the same coin. To help restrict calories and offset some of the undesirable weight gained by over-indulging, some resort to deprivation in other moments as the answer. This approach is as treacherous as quick-sand. Not only does it increase your susceptibility to willpower fatigue, but it can also lead to malnutrition, which ultimately affects all systems in the body.

Both hypoglycemia (low blood sugar) and hyper-glycemia (high blood sugar) impair your ability to sus-tain balanced emotions and clear thinking. If blood glucose is too low, your brain cues the liver to make more glucose. It does this by sending a distress signal to trigger the release of the stress hormone epinephrine (adrenaline). Unlike the imaginary scenarios that play themselves in a loop in our minds, low blood sugar is a real, identifiable threat that should be avoided. With that said, periodic fasting and detoxification can be ben-eficial to our health in some instances; but it is nei-ther a viable nor safe means of maintaining or reducing body weight over the long-term. Self-inflicted famine can be considered as abusive to oneself, and I strongly advise against using it as a method of controlling emo-tional eating.

Let's revisit our garden again with this greater understanding. Each of our thoughts and beliefs can be compared to little magical seeds. With enough attention, nurturing, and tending to those seeds, each one of them has the ability to reveal itself in your garden as some form of a plant. So think of our actions, behaviours, and habits as the harvest that's grown from these seeds. What we produce in our life as a result of those actions can be likened to the fruits that have been cultivated.

Imagine the compulsion to reach out for food as an undesirable weed that has revealed itself in the garden. The infestation of these weeds competes with the crops of the fruits, stealing their resources and making them vulnerable to risk. Of course, the toxic plant needs to be removed, but focusing on quitting the action itself is like cutting the plant from its stem and expecting that it won't come back. In reality, we know that method has one impending fate. The weeds will return. At the root of this plant is a feeling, one or more emotional dependencies. To successfully transform the state of your personal garden, the focus must shift away from targeting the plant itself. Rather, the goal should be focusing on pruning the root of the emotion while planting new, more desirable seeds.

Planting seeds of love and admiration is absolutely a must, but yanking destructive roots is equally important. No real change can be made until one recognizes both the feeling at the root and which seed (core belief or thought) is continually being planted and nurtured that is leading to the infestation of the garden. Without that insight, combined with dedication towards pruning out the old and planting the new, the survival of the entire garden is at risk.

Our emotional states are influenced by our lifestyle choices, but changing our lifestyle (eating habits) is subject to our emotional states. Addressing our lifestyle choices without addressing our feelings only transfers the addiction to some other thing.

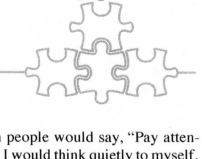

CHAPTER 10

Attention

I used to detest it when people would say, "Pay attention to your thoughts." I would think quietly to myself, *As if I could do that. Do you have any idea how many thoughts are speeding through my mind all day? How is anyone meant to monitor all those thoughts?* It seemed absurd and vastly unobtainable.

However, what was really absurd was that for a great length of time, I never fully grasped the power of this invaluable piece of advice. While it's true that we have a multitude of thoughts floating in and out of our minds each day, many of those thoughts are quite similar. A great deal of the thoughts you have today are comparable to the thoughts you had yesterday. Yesterday's program ran as a sequel to the day before, and so on. Paying attention to what's being constantly broadcasted through your mind gives the insight as to what paradigm you've become trapped inside.

A paradigm is a framework enclosing ways of thinking, basic assumptions, and methodology that are accepted and thus serve as a model. Entire families and societies can live within the bounds of a specific paradigm, but each individual can also be detained by their own personal paradigm as well. If you are stuck in a subconscious pattern of thinking, doing, and being, then you are in fact living within the confinements of your own self-imposed paradigm—one that has been positioned solely by your beliefs and perceptions.

The subconscious mind can be programmed to operate within the bounds of whatever paradigm we choose. Both our reality and our state of being are the end-products of what we have conditioned the subconscious mind to express.

While our conscious mind is interpreting an infinitesimal fraction of the environmental stimuli around us at any given moment, our subconscious is processing 500,000 times more stimuli than the conscious mind. Just as you don't have to consciously instruct yourself to breathe, you don't have to consciously instruct yourself to play out the character that you have become accustomed to being. In reality, your conscious mind has dominion over both, but it can't process nearly as much information as your subconscious. This means any belief, thought accompanied with emotion, or behaviour that is rehearsed several times by your conscious mind can eventually be learned by the subconscious, and then be set as an automatic program that your consciousness no longer has to think about to sustain. This can make us more efficient by freeing the consciousness up to process other things, such as new information and/or experiences.

Our most common thoughts, actions, and behaviours become nondeclarative memories (implicit memories) run by the subconscious mind (also known as unconscious mind). The rule is, therefore, survival of the busiest thoughts.

128

If you think about it, not only are your thoughts today almost identical to the ones you had yesterday, so are most of your behaviours and reactions. Essentially, we spend a great deal of our time behaving in our own specific pattern that is no different than the day before. Each of your actions can not only be triggered by your environment, but also by the thoughts you have conditioned yourself to repeat. Reconditioning the body also means reconstructing the paradigm we are imprisoned in.

In order for your mind to expand, the conscious mind needs to be open and exposed to novel and meaningful things. Once new and relevant information is absorbed through repetition or elevated emotion, it can be memorized.

The greater the attention your brain pays to a given stimulus, the more data will be learned and encrypted. To survive in the wild, it was imperative that we learn from our mistakes; it was critical to pay attention to particular things at the expense of others. As a result of this awareness, we create memories and learn in a particular way. Our attention then governs our learning. As we know, our attention is ruled by our emotions, beliefs, and desires.

The brain takes more notice when exposed to new and meaningful things. This is why children struggle to grasp concepts about information they don't really care about in school; they have not linked how the information they are being taught serves their personal goals at that stage of their life, resulting in little to no retention. Any data that makes its way through the gates of their mind in the brief moments when they try and pay attention is not perceived as valuable to their current existence. They are neither emotionally stimulated by it, nor do they retrieve the data enough times to store it; thus, nothing is memorized.

Now, if you are cemented in a circuit of feeling, thinking, and doing the same things within the framework of your specific paradigm, you risk being unexposed to a novel stimulus. Therefore, every day is a continuum of the previous day, performing the same routine actions, going to the same places, talking about the same things with the same people, exposing yourself to the same boring stimuli day after day. It's no wonder one would desire a stimulant. In this particular case, we look for that stimulant in the kitchen. Our paradigm restriction stands starkly in the way of new learning and wipes out any chance of establishing new implicit memories (also known as habits).

In order for the mind to expand in a new direction, it needs to be challenged with a new emotionally valuable stimulus. Let's not forget how our good friend dopamine causes us to narrow our focus and facilitates new learning; simply exposing yourself to new emotionally valuable information raises your levels of dopamine, causing you to pay attention, leading to new learning, and can also reinforce the desire to continue to expand in that new direction. The mundane does none of these great things.

We need something natural to raise our dopamine levels. We are designed to desire so that we can move forward and expand. When we are stuck in an unstimulating routine, we inevitably begin to depend on substances such as food to energize the senses and raise our levels of dopamine. Failing to step out into new territory fences in the growth of the mind, which fundamentally impacts the integrity of your entire garden.

Until you recognize the patterns of the paradigm you are currently living in, you can't accurately determine what you need to change. In other words, you have trouble getting unstuck because you can't recognize what it is that has boxed you in. One stray thought can be enough to slip you back into the same old patterns.

Making a lasting change means rehearsing new thoughts and behaviours with greater frequency than the old thoughts and behaviours, while simultaneously altering the internal chemistry to feel a new emotional state. Differentiating between the old and new program requires you to pay attention to your busiest thoughts now so you can become familiar with the old program's characteristics. You can then use this insight to determine if you are operating from the old, outdated paradigm, or within the desired new future paradigm. If you recognize that you have slipped back into the old agenda, you can use your consciousness to take the necessary steps to change it. (I will provide techniques to do this in a later chapter.) If you do this consistently, you will eventually find yourself adopting new habits of thinking, feeling, and being.

As you see, we can't just wish to be a new person with new habits and then lay back and hope we become that person. We must consciously act like we already are that new desired person by thinking thoughts that are in alignment with our new desired paradigm. While making sure that these new thoughts are the busiest of all our thoughts, we have to simultaneously alter our emotional chemistry. And if combined with repetition of new routines, we can invoke the subconscious to create memories stemming from our new patterns.

New territory is unknown, and the unknown possesses both great risks and great rewards. Feeling scared and excited is a good indicator that you have just stepped outside of your comfort zone and are now in the process of potentially creating some kind of change. Scared and excited means expansion. Although stepping outside of your paradigm can feel initially unsettling, it is essential to experience it if personal advancement is the goal. You have to get comfortable with strategically making yourself uncomfortable. With time, your comfort zone can expand, new habits can form, and you can find yourself operating within the framework of an altered paradigm.

Unfortunately, without conscious awareness, it is very easy for the unconscious mind to lure you back into the cage of the old paradigm. Anxieties can effortlessly seduce you right back into your comfort zone, where the unconscious can blissfully operate based on what it knows and what it's been conditioned to be most comfortable with. At times like these, what can often happen is that frightening thoughts begin to take up more of your attention, rather than the exciting, opportunistic thoughts you started out with. A new emotional state is not generated within the body, nor is it rehearsed with greater frequency than the old, negative emotional state, meaning that if a significant alteration to the internal habit was not created, the subconscious mind doesn't change either. Willpower ultimately lags; the individual gets spooked and is steered right back into their comfort zone to resume life as usual. We refer to this process as *self-sabotage*.

Unbeknownst to the conscious mind, the subconscious drives you right back to wherever you have conditioned it to take you. The destination your subconscious believes it should take you to is based on its records of past events and not on your unlimited potentials in the future—unless, of course, you teach it otherwise. The subconscious is much like a supercomputer that has the ability to download infinite potential programs. It only operates within the program it has already downloaded until it has been conditioned to download a new program. You can now appreciate how invaluable your conscious awareness really is, and how precious it is to truly know thyself. As promised, I will uncover more strategies on how to do that in the ensuing chapters.

To pay attention means to take notice, to become aware, and to direct focus. Most of us are familiar with the statement, "What you focus on, grows." Yet for a great deal of my life, I paid the most attention to what I *didn't* want, as opposed to what I wanted to create. As you can imagine, not only did I get more of what I didn't want, it also consumed all of my attention. Failing to understand the wisdom in that adage was one of the main sources of my misery.

I guess I kind of understood it, in the simplest of terms. If I focused on something, over time, it'll grow. Yeah, sure, got it (insert eye roll). I didn't really acknowledge that everything—your addictions, your limitations, your daily stresses, your beliefs, and your anxieties—all need to be included in that adage.

I refused to appreciate that my focus was a powerful force and that my awareness governed my entire personal reality—both externally and internally. I certainly had no concept that it was my beliefs and emotions that directed my attention. I stopped dead in my tracks when I realized that we are like little magicians that can convert the energetic force that runs through us to create anything we desire. We have the power to direct our energy with our focus and transform it through our intentions.

The law of conservation of energy states that "energy can never be created or destroyed; it can only be transformed." When you are depleting your personal energy reserves to expend energy on a problem, a person, or a thought of what you don't want, none of that energy is lost; it simply becomes transformed. So, it makes sense that the degree to which we focus on a problem determines the abundance of energetic accelerant it receives and how powerful it becomes in our lives. There is a truly magnificent life force energy that is available within all of us, and we have the capacity to use our focus to direct it to our choosing.

Let's travel back to that moment when we are standing in front of the mirror chanting all our affirmations. Through years of conditioning, simply looking in the direction of a mirror triggered me to instantly focus on my perceived physical shortcomings. I criticized myself in front of a mirror and felt the negative emotions associated with those fault-finding thoughts on so many occasions that the act became a force of habit. I'm certain that there are many who share in this vicious habit. I like to describe negative body image as though it's a psychological cancer that has spread throughout society with its roots so embedded in the paradigm of what society believes beauty looks like.

Through repetition and emotional charge, the mirror itself can simply become a cue that automatically prompts us to focus on our perceived physical imperfections, while remaining visionless to any of our other assets. Because nerve cells that fire together, wire together, the mirror and negative emotion can become linked. Even anticipating looking at your reflection can prepare you to pay attention to these shortcomings once you arrive in front of the mirror.

Remember, simply the anticipation of walking through my front door was a trigger that spurred me to start planning what I would eat when I got home. Anticipating looking in the mirror can also cue negative thoughts and beliefs. These strong but deeply incorrect concepts are all nothing but subconscious programs of thinking, feeling, and reacting, and have no basis on reality. Allowing our focus to be directed merely by habit excludes us from being able to collect data from the bigger picture. Everything we experience is little more than an illusion.

Despite the new words you are now saying, if the emotional elixir inside doesn't change, then it's likely that no significant impact will be made. If you list your affirmations, but actually have an old, opposing, subconscious belief or attitude about yourself, then your emotional state will be congruent with the old belief. If no new emotion is generated, then new learning won't take place. In other words, if you don't feel like the new person, you won't ever become that new person.

Listing affirmations, without also rehearsing what it feels like to be that person, means that you are not being—you are simply trying. Trying implies striving for a goal, but you don't strive to be the person you

135

already believe that you are. You believe that the person you are is just the reality, so you just do. If you are well and healthy, you don't try to get up every morning and try to brush your teeth. You do not imagine all the potential obstacles that might get in the way of your routine. Nor do you attempt to make it to work; you simply get up, perform your everyday routine, and you just make it there. Very little gets in the way of a goal once it has been converted into a pattern and has become a way of being.

When one tries, they hold the belief that something could stop them; but if an individual makes the decision to *do*, they hold a belief that their actions are certain to lead to a specific outcome. Trying implies that you have not fully embodied it. To reprogram the mind and body, you absolutely have to personify the character of the kind of person who would obtain the specific goal they desire. That includes beliefs, emotions, perceptions, thoughts, and behaviours. This is why addressing these areas is at the core of my 90-day program, "The Eating Enigma: 90 days to transforming your relationship with food." Your desires need to be backed by an empowering belief; otherwise, nothing comes of them. Without faith, your desires are never realized, just as their physical counterparts can never become a reality. In other words, your desires don't manifest because the subconscious is operating an opposing program, and all of your unconscious decisions are made with the intention of manifesting an opposing reality.

Cognitive dissonance describes the tension that's experienced by a person who simultaneously holds two or more contradictory beliefs when carrying forth an action that contradicts those beliefs or when confronted with data that contradicts existing beliefs. Some examples are: one might believe that eating healthy is good for the body, but also holds the belief that eating healthy means you might be ridiculed and dubbed a hippie or health nut. Or, perhaps one believes that their quality of life would improve if they could lose weight, but they may also hold a contrary belief that losing weight means that they will be subscribing to a life devoid of pleasures. Alternatively, a person can believe that eating well is important, but it's expensive to eat healthy, and their cravings are more powerful than their will, so they believe they can neither afford it nor have the will to overcome cravings. A final example is this: one may believe they can build wealth, but also carry the belief that money is the root of all evil. In the case of cognitive dissonance, we sabotage one goal at the expense of another, even if we aren't consciously aware that the latter is also one of our goals.

When listing positive affirmations, the momentary feeling of discomfort that sometimes emerges is a sure signal that what you are saying is in contradiction with an old and limiting belief. That outdated belief doesn't reveal the truth about your unlimited potential; it only announces what you have chosen to believe. The conscious mind can hold the awareness that the old belief is irrational and is based on the perceptions of only a few past experiences, but if the unconscious has failed to be reprogrammed by the conscious, the stronger of the two beliefs wins. Beliefs that trigger the most frightening thoughts and emotions will force the individual to forfeit the opposing beliefs and goals, unless, of course, the individual chooses to apply the force of love. Love is the only emotion that trumps fear.

In Chapter 4, you performed an exercise where I asked you to list the excuses for why you believed you haven't already achieved your goals. Those rationalizations provided you with insight on some of your limiting beliefs. I also pointed out that those excuses didn't apply to the goals you believed you could attain, and consequently had obtained. Those limiting beliefs held no value when you loved yourself enough to believe that goal was destined for you, or if you loved an idea enough to go after it. The excuses only took precedence when you believed you didn't deserve to obtain a particular goal, or that trying would prove to be less rewarding than if you put aside your excuses and went for it.

Adaptation takes place when the organism finds itself in a new environment. Remember, real or imagined, the brain doesn't know the difference. Nightmares, fantasies, dreams, or reality — if you feel an elevated emotion, then a physiological change to the internal habit has been created. We must exercise both will and faith to embody a change in order for the change to become hardwired in the brain. Real change requires you to use your will to produce new thoughts and evoke new feelings, so you feel like the change has already occurred. It also causes you to take action over and over again in a new direction while holding onto unshakable faith. This can create just enough of an internal shift for your subconscious to update its program. Once you reach that threshold where the two minds are in alignment, the conscious mind can surrender its will. The subconscious can take over to maintain the new state of being.

This infinite intelligence that lives within all of us processes billions of bits of information every single moment. It orchestrates your entire reality, from regulating your immune system to making sure you walk with your left foot in front of your right, and so forth. Your conscious mind doesn't have to worry about pumping your blood through your veins because of this wisdom that's within all of us. Some of the processes the unconscious sustains are innate, and some are learned through experience and repetition. Once this wisdom begins to exert its will towards your goals, the conscious mind can move on to work on the next illusion. At this stage, the conscious mind no longer has to worry about how — it just has to continue to believe that the intelligence will.

Paying attention to your thoughts gives you insight into what you actually believe now, and what current paradigm you are operating in. You can stand in front of a mirror and say, "I'm healthy," all you want, but if your belief suggests otherwise, then the majority of your thoughts will too, and that will be reflected in your lifestyle. Affirmations are only influential when belief and emotion are combined. When practiced in this effective manner, there is little that is more powerful than verbal persuasion.

Faith is having certainty in someone or something despite whether it has yet to materialise or not. We have the liberty to exercise our will to accept, believe, and surrender to anything. We can have free will to hold faith on any possibility. Faith has the capacity to generate emotions so powerful they make a change to the internal environment, despite what's going on in the external world. Being loyal to an outcome before it materialises suggests you have faith in the outcome.

This is where I'd like to invite gratitude to take center stage. Feeling grateful for a future experience that you've chosen to have faith in, instead of focusing on the resentments of your past experiences, and repeating that practice over and over again, shifts the paradigm you live in. You will evolve in whichever direction you're most focused on and exercise most frequently. Surrogacy can not only be applied to your actions in the midst of a craving, but is also a profitable practice when used to amend your thoughts and beliefs.

It is not powerful enough to solely lean on surrogacy during the allotted time that you are listing your affirmations while you simultaneously spend the rest of the day operating in the framework of an outdated paradigm that's based on old beliefs. Any time your awareness tunes in and acknowledges that you have wandered off and are functioning within the limitations of old, habitual thoughts and emotions, detach from those thoughts and focus on a surrogate thought instead. It is crucial to ensure that the surrogate thoughts you have chosen and the emotions they awaken are in alignment with your new goals.

What is the mind doing in the moments when we aren't paying attention? What is it focusing on?

Well, we know novel and meaningful cognitive activities cause you to activate your executive brain, making you pay attention to the present moment. When we are in familiar and mundane territory and running on autopilot, the executive brain is at rest, but the other parts of your brain are very active. When the mind wanders, we are spending time in a highly active default baseline state. This state is known as *default mode network* (DMN). When you are staying present, you are less likely to slip into DMN.

We are constantly shifting between maintaining focused awareness on the environment and reverie, or daydreaming, if you will. When we are ruminating, we have drifted into DMN. It's a normal process that occurs for everyone. DMN isn't inherently good or bad; it can prove to be useful for creativity and reflecting upon new stimulus.

When we are in DMN, we revert to our default baseline state and operate based on our habits. Even if the conscious mind is unaware, the subconscious is simultaneously tuning into millions of signals being received from our environment. Those signals trigger habitual thoughts, emotions, cravings, and finally, behaviours. In DMN, most if not all our unoriginal thoughts are being cued through mere force of habit. Because your subconscious can tune into signals that can easily go undetected by the conscious mind, such as subliminal messages in adverts and various other stimuli all around us, I can't stress the importance enough to be aware of all of your triggers.

Thinking about thinking is known as *metacognition*. The term metacognition literally means cognition about cognition. In practice, we can use metacognition to self-regulate our own thoughts and raise our self-awareness. It is a gift that is instrumental to mastering our own lives. Cravings are a blessing in disguise, because when you have drifted off in DMN, your cravings can alert your conscious mind that your thoughts wandered off into the old paradigm. If you view cravings as opportunities to pay attention to your thoughts and further change them—instead of interpreting them as a curse—then they are no longer working against you, but are now working for you. You can assume your rightful position as the master, and the cravings are no more than your slave.

Let your cravings be an alarm that alerts you to pay attention to whatever you were just thinking. Your impulsive habits—contrary to what you have always believed—can work for you if you know the secrets on how to use them, which you now do. Silencing the alarm by giving into the craving doesn't abate the problem. It is no different than ripping the smoke detector off the ceiling, then watching the entire building burn down. Pay attention, and then take the necessary steps to put out the fire while creating a new routine that ultimately leads to the core need or reward you are actually seeking.

In the midst of a craving, there is one vital thing to remember: you have now slipped into one of your automatic programs, which is likely to lead you into the old paradigm you are trying to escape from. The most empowering thing to keep in mind at this stage is that you are not your thoughts; you are simply the observer of these thoughts. Some of the most dangerous things one can do at this time is get caught up in these thoughts; argue or reason with these thoughts; or let these thoughts convince you that they know what's best for you. Most, if not all, of the thoughts that are triggered during a craving are simply what I call the *automatic, self-sabotaging, addictive voice* at play. This voice has no control over your actions; it merely presents a convincing case that you have not only heard many times before, but have also given in to time and time again.

There are two types of thoughts your executive brain will need to observe and override.

1. Any thought(s) or belief(s) that may have been the cue that initially spurred the craving.
2. Any thought(s) or belief(s) that tries to steer you back into the old paradigm by convincing you it's a good idea to do so.

All of these thoughts will have one thing in common; they will sound very familiar. The thoughts in the second category are usually only convincing to you once you have been triggered by one of your cues, but they tend not bear weight at any other time. In fact, when you reflect on them in the moments when you aren't having a craving, you may wonder how they ever convinced you to give in. They are thoughts that sound like these:

- I have been good, so this week, I deserve a treat.
- One bite isn't going to hurt me; I've learned self-control.
- I have already cheated today; I might as well make a day of it.
- I have had a bad day; I deserve this.
- I don't care about my goals. I feel like having this, so I am going to have it.
- Everything in moderation.
- I'm too busy for this. I don't have the time to find a healthy option.
- This is ridiculous; I'm going to eat what I want.

The most persistent and convincing of these thoughts will be the ones you happen to have given in to the most frequently in the past. This is simply the subconscious operating within the program it has downloaded from the past through repetition and elevated emotion.

What often happens in the case of an unhealthy relationship with food is the individual will initially try to fight the craving by arguing or reasoning with the automatic, self-sabotaging, addictive voice. This inner dialogue naturally begins to cause internal tension that ultimately can only be relieved by eating.

Yet, there is no need to engage with the outdated program; the addictive voice is only that—a voice. It has absolutely no ability to control your actions. It only holds the capacity to hypnotically lure you to choose to take a particular route. In other words, the voice itself holds no power if you choose not to engage with it. As the observer, you are 100 percent in control over how much time you spend listening to its case.

Imagine your garden again. We know that the emotional addiction can be compared to an infestation that has gone beyond your control (or so you had believed). Your focus on the infestation is what is connecting it to its only true energy supply. To shift your attention is to cut the cord that your emotional addiction uses to feed. Every time you allow yourself to repeat a particular thought, it's like a vote for what gets to grow inside your mind, even if it's a weed. It's not the garden that we have been granted that is the villain or the hero in our stories. What determines its health and vitality is more closely connected to the quality of the force and the intention that runs through it; that's what truly needs examining.

CHAPTER 11

Inspiration

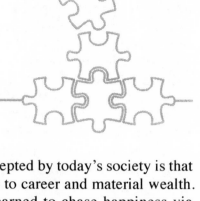

The toxic delusion accepted by today's society is that success equates only to career and material wealth. We have, in essence, learned to chase happiness via things. When the novelty of the new flavour of ice cream, new outfit, new car, or new home wears off, we are still left feeling uneasy. What many of us fail to notice is that the desire to reach for these goals is a desperate attempt at obtaining some sort of security; unfortunately for us, the attempts are futile, because nothing in the material world is secure. We have exaggerated the value of material possessions at the expense of our wellbeing. When we finish eating the chocolate cake, or the excitement of the new relationship wears off, we are left only with the same feelings that initially pushed us to pursue these goals.

Now, I am not saying that life isn't much more comfortable when we have enjoyable careers and some freedom due to wealth. In fact, I am a firm believer that a fulfilling vocation and general wellbeing are very much linked. Having the financial resources to live according to what is valuable to us contributes significantly to our wellbeing. We should absolutely be very grateful for these things if we are fortunate enough to have them. If it's inspiring for you to go after something, then by all means, go for the gold. I am simply pointing out that if the desire to obtain these goals is with the intention to secure something that you perceive will bring you peace, then that reveals your current emotional set point is not set at peace. No physical reward—chocolate included—will give us that peace for an extended length of time. The idea of "I will be at peace when..." is an indication you are not already at peace. You are, in actuality, chasing an illusion. Thus we find ourselves in this predictable rat race where we need more of the stimulus each and every time we have an urge.

I may have confused you a little here, because all along I have encouraged you to set goals. I have explained the significance of having a goal and serving a purpose here on earth, as it relates to your recovery. I've illustrated how a life devoid of a mission puts you at risk for seeking dopamine in potentially toxic things. Now I am advising that you not seek happiness by setting a goal to chase things.

The truth is, we do need goals. We need to continually strive to move forward. Making consistent progress is exceedingly important. Everything in nature is either growing, or it is dying. Growth is essential to our vitality. The intention behind our goals is what matters the most. If the goal you are seeking is with the intention of reaching an elevated emotion, then the reward will always be fleeting.

The fuel you use to propel yourself forward makes a difference to the potential outcomes you yield. The primary life force energy that you choose to shine over your garden is the significant difference between producing wholesome fruits, poisonous fruits, or worse yet, no fruits at all.

Our intentions can be either from a place of motivation or from a place of inspiration, and there is a place for both. When we are designing our own life and setting goals for our future, the best intention is inspiration. Operating from a place of motivation when it's time for inspiration to step in is where we run into trouble. I promise I will explain how I differentiate between the two, but first, we need to discuss fear.

Moving forward and propelling yourself ahead is going to be both exciting and fearful at times, because both are linked to the unknown. If we want to grow, we need to take steps into the unknown, which invites with it the potential of feeling strong emotions from either side of the spectrum. Even when we don't want to grow, we simply cannot avoid stepping into the new. The only thing that is truly ever constant in this world is change. Fear is inevitable.

But don't worry; what I am sharing with you has nothing to do with facing your fears. We've become familiar with the statement, "What you focus on, grows," so it would be of no value to you that I suggest focusing on battling fear itself. What I am asking is that you honour your desires by taking action steps towards them despite your anxieties. What I aim to be doing is quite simply merging some scientific data with encouraging words in the hopes that I might entice you to see the benefits to your life in making your own change. We've already discussed how everything we choose to do is a direct result of a perceived benefit to do it, and I'm delivering this information with the hopes that the more you learn about the magnificence of your mind, body, and all of Mother Nature combined, the more likely you'll be willing to choose to do whatever it takes to care for them all. What I'm advocating is the idea of expressing this love by doing things that inspire you, while also creating something of service in this world.

In order for me to accurately explain how I differentiate between motivation and inspiration, I need to first make a distinction between fear and anxiety. There is a significant variance between the two. While both can use similar pathways in the brain, and the feelings they generate within the body resemble one another, they are, in fact, very different.

When you are presented with an immediate, identifiable threat, it is the fear response that has the potential to save you. Sitting in lotus pose recounting your affirmations while a lion is making its way towards you is stupid. If we didn't have fear, then we would do these types of ridiculous things.

Much to the dismay of positive thinkers, fear is never going anywhere. As much as we love to blame something, fear does not get in the way of our dreams, either. In fact, it serves our mission in the sense that it keeps us alive long enough that we can go after them. You and I would be long dead if it weren't for our fear. We can be sure that if it didn't serve a purpose to our existence, then Mother Nature would have wiped it out many years ago—just as she has done and will continue to do with everything else (us included). Fear has its place and we should be grateful for it. Despite how much we have villainized it, it is actually our friend.

Fear is when your awareness acknowledges that there is a hazard in your immediate environment or that you are currently at risk of encountering a real threat.

It signals and prepares your body to either fight or flee from the predator or prey. The mind instantaneously assesses the risks and rewards, and then your body swiftly reacts. Fear is awesome. We are programmed to feel fear when faced with the unknown, to proceed with caution, and to use our senses to pay attention to potential risks. Fear makes us alert. The unknown spawns a list of possible new dangers that we need to be aware of and account for.

There are two basic types of fear.

1. Fear of something that has come into your life and puts your survival at risk. This is the fear that we have gained some form of predator.
2. Fear of the loss of something that you perceive to be critical to your survival. This is the fear that you may lose some form of prey.

Fear is a basic instinct. When our lives, and the things in our lives that we value the most, are truly at risk, survival mode is paramount. Fear is Survival 101. Fear mode is spectacular when there is truly something to fear.

Anxiety, however, is different. It is inauthentic, and making the choice to listen to it is tantamount to subscribing to lies. Anxiety is when there is no present danger, but your thoughts are convincing your body that you're at risk. Imagining some future event while pondering the risks of something that has not yet occurred (and is statistically unlikely to happen the way you imagined), is anxiety. When you are presently safe, but your body is operating in survival mode, that is not you being fearful; that is you being anxious.

Perpetual anxiety is a great indicator that you may have developed an emotional dependency on fear. It means you are often operating from the stress response and, consequently, you are just simply surviving. Excessive anxiety is like a pernicious vine that strangles your dreams, wraps them in "what if?" and chokes them with "I could never!" It is merciless, volatile, and infamous for murdering our life's mission.

Both fear and anxiety are incredibly motivating. Embrace fear. When you are in serious trouble, let it consume you; let it possess your thoughts and allow it to move you. You're as good as dead without it. Anxiety, on the other hand, you don't need so much—although some anxiety is normal. When the operating system you are working in is fear-based, you are making decisions from motivation. It would be ludicrous to look at the lion and say, "Excuse me, I am inspired to sit here and chant right now. Do you want to join me?" No, you would make a move!

Motivation is influenced by something outside of you. Whether it be a predator or prey, something makes you move. In some instances, it can cause you to freeze. But in any case, environmental factors have influenced your decisions. Some external influence has sparked an emotion which has set the body in motion. When an outside influence has pushed you to do something, it is motivation, and it's always survival mode.

When you believe you should act in a given manner so that people will like you, you are being motivated to do that thing. When you believe you should look or act a certain way to find love, you are being motivated to behave that way. When you take a job because it would make your mother happy, you are being motivated to take the job.

If our default baseline state is at peace, then whenever there isn't an immediate danger present, we should be in rest and relaxation (PNS). In PNS, we are thriving. Decisions made from this place can be made from inspiration.

Motivation, although vital when we are in danger, is based from either fear or anxiety. The intention is to not lose that which you have deemed most crucial to your survival, or to not gain something that puts your survival at risk.

Inspiration is when our mind surrenders its will to the internal compass so it can lead the way. When we trust in the wisdom within us that knows what's best for us, we are being inspired. In other words, by doing things because we have a keen interest in them, or simply because they are meaningful to us, that is acting from a place of inspiration—and that's my definition of thriving. The reward is self-satisfaction, and it's the most delicious of them all.

We all have something that is meaningful to us; we just feel inspired to have it in our life. Typically, it's something that we are naturally good at or we feel compelled to learn more about. We often wish we had more time to engage in it. We don't quite understand why, but we find it incredibly fascinating. I'll give you a hint—it's not that thing that you keep procrastinating to do. Nobody has to push you to get up out of bed to go do it. You have three main resources—time, energy, and money. It doesn't bother you to spend any of your resources on it. You find yourself running late for things because of it, and you're willing to expend energy working on it, even if you don't have to. You find yourself speaking about it often with others. You might even call in sick to work so you can be with it. When a dollar comes into your life, you invest a great deal of the dollar towards it.

Believe it or not, your current life reveals what you are inspired by. It's very difficult for anxiety to keep it completely out of your world. It is magnetic, and there is a pull that draws you towards it. Despite anxiety's greatest efforts, it has in some capacity made its way into your life. Anxiety just makes sure you don't master it enough that you go empower yourself with it. It would never stand for that! Anxiety brainwashes you by saying whatever it needs to say to convince you that you are not destined for greatness, and that it should lead the way. Its case is convincing, its voice is hypnotic, and its dialogue sounds something like this...

- "What will people say if I fail?"
- "What will my parents think of that?"
- "What if I make a mistake and it doesn't work out?"
- "I am too old; people will laugh at me."
- "I would never make money doing that!"
- "There's no point; I am not lucky enough for it to work out."
- "I couldn't imagine myself doing that."
- "I am not talented enough."
- "Did I turn the stove off?"
- "What if I lose all of my money trying it?"
- "What if my partner leaves me because of it?"
- "I am not smart enough; what if I do something stupid?"

- "I don't know how."
- "Did I turn the stove off?"
- "What if I gain all my weight back?"
- "I don't have the skills that my next-door neighbour has, and I need to be more like him to be successful."
- "I've never been popular, so no one will want what I have to offer."
- "This is a crazy idea."
- "I have children; I can't start a new career."
- "Did I turn the stove off?"
- "I can't do anything right."
- "Maybe it's in my best interest not to try."
- "I never finish anything anyway."
- "I should drive back home and double check the stove."

The seeds of anxiety are the shrieking words of worry and doubt.

There are different degrees of anxiety. Some are riddled with anxious thoughts, while others tend to be more affected by specific things. Now, some anxiety is normal. We all experience it sometimes. However, when anxiety hijacks our will to live an inspired life, mutes our creative expression, and influences the perceptions of our natural-born gifts, it becomes a liability to our wellbeing that we should have no tolerance for.

Whereas inspiration sounds a bit more like this...

- "Oh, that's interesting; let me try that."
- "I think the world could use this; let me give it to them."
- "I'd like to make this...I am going to do it."

- "I don't know how yet, but I'm going to learn."
- "That was a good lesson; I'll do it better next time."
- "I deserve to be successful with my special talents, as much as my neighbour deserves to be successful with his."
- "I could do that."
- "I'm so glad I am finally seeing progress; I can't wait to see how much further I go."
- "I'm going to keep moving forward; this is fun."
- "I still really love this; I'm going to stick with this, even when it gets hard."
- "This is challenging, but so meaningful to me; I am glad I am doing it."
- "I'm not sure how, but I'm sure I'll just figure it out along the way."

The seeds of inspiration are the whispers of truthful and loving thoughts.

At this stage, I could claim that once you have uncovered what you have been put on this earth to do, then nothing but magic will fill your universe. Every door of opportunity will burst open for you, and at the end of your struggle, there will be nothing but a pot of gold waiting for you. But I would be blatantly lying and selling you nothing more than another fantasy.

Selling fantasies doesn't get you results. All it does is get you to waste your time and energy chasing something that simply doesn't exist anywhere on earth — except maybe in the movies. Believing in a mistruth and expecting the universe to live outside of its own laws is as corrupt and unjust as it is to not live according to your own truth. It shifts the focus from that which is

154

attainable (your mission) to that which has never been obtained (support without challenge). It sets us up to feel incredibly let down in the process.

I acknowledge that this is where you might not like me so much, but my end goal here has less to do with me being liked and more to do with me being an integral part of your genuine healing. So, with that goal in mind, I'm willing to put myself at risk for not being so popular by being authentic and sincere. I know I started this story with, "Once upon a time," but I am going to be completely candid with you. It's not going to end with ". . . happily ever after." This is because I am obsessed with real facts, and they show that there's no such thing as a fairy-tale ending, at least so far. Pretending that there is a stage in life where we will obtain only support without challenge, light without darkness, push without pull, elation without depression, or even excitement without fear, sets us up for nothing but resentment and resistance to the truth about our harmonious universe.

If you are doing things for the personal satisfaction of doing them, the natural ebbs and flows of life along the journey won't impact you so much, because you are not as attached to a perceived life-or-death outcome. Rather, it's simply for the thrill of doing it, and subsequent further learning about it that becomes the real journey; it's the journey itself that is the treat. When you are doing something for the sake of your survival, then adversity could trigger you to erupt. Rewards from motivation are not nearly as satiating as rewards from inspiration. You'll always feel like there is something missing; fulfillment will elude you, and you'll feel as though something isn't quite right. Eventually that feeling overcomes us, and we search for the cure in the fridge.

The truth is, I have no idea what the outcome will be for you when you follow your heart. But on the bright side, neither do you. Obsessively indulging in the risk-versus-rewards game of future potential is a waste of time. This is simply because there is no way to foretell which of the risks and rewards are certain to reveal themselves in the future.

In the case of a real, identifiable threat, the ability to weigh the costs versus benefits helps us determine if it's optimal to run, attack, or freeze. You can rely on your instincts in that moment. The future is a mystery. There is no way to calculate the drawbacks and advantages effectively if you can't also foresee which of the potentials are guaranteed to manifest themselves. Over-contemplating the ideas you are inspired to do puts your true personal potential at risk against the imaginary personal limitations you have set in your mind.

Anything can inspire you. You can feel inspired to create wealth. Some people just love the stock markets, and they enjoy investing their money in building wealth. Health and wellness could be an interest. You could feel called to learn about astrology. Writing a book could be a burning desire. Social status could just naturally be a high priority for you. We often discount what we know we want because we think we should want the same things that other people want. In reality, we are each perfectly designed vessels that can bring into the world whatever we feel called to create. We are here to express ourselves through our own unique gifts.

I believe we all have many gifts inside us, waiting to be found. We have the will to choose from whatever gifts have been divinely given to us. We build on and refine our natural-born gifts by learning about them, applying ourselves, and mastering them. Don't compare your talents and creative expressions to anyone else. Imagine the tragedy to the wine industry if the grape vineyard looked over at the apricot orchard and decided, "I am not doing this right." Remember, Mother Nature doesn't seem to allow for anything that doesn't serve a purpose. If you are here, it's for a unique reason. You are not her only mistake in the history of time. Despite what anxiety desperately wants to convince us of, you and I are just as magnificent as everything else that Mother Nature creates.

CHAPTER 12

Permission

M any of us search our entire lifetime for some meaning in our lives. We have the tendency to wait for people, events, and experiences to make us feel worthy of just being alive. We put limitations on how far we can go in our future based on where we have been in the past. Think of it like this; before we are willing to see our own greatness, we wait for some cryptic sign telling us that we are, in fact, great. We fail to acknowledge the fact that we were even born as a definite sign of greatness. We let our perceived failures characterize us for life and subsequently attach ambiguous meaning to traumas, resulting in us living our lives according to what we have decided is meant for us. Our current environment is somehow allowed to determine how great our future potential can be. We expend our most precious commodity—time—by simply waiting for something to give us permission to be who we naturally are. When you have the courage to take your emotional goggles off, even for a moment, you would bear witness to the evidence of this permission every time you take in a breath.

I believe that we all share a few things in common. We long to love, be loved, and we yearn for a meaning to our life. Without some kind of direction or target to obtain, we lack the necessary dopamine we need to feel enthusiastic and alive. To love, be loved, and to have a sense of purpose, all help to provide us with the necessary neurochemistry we need.

It is an unfortunate fact that the fate for many of us is to turn to food as our main source of reward. The only way to break a toxic love affair with food is to focus your love somewhere else. It is a necessity to desire something more. In order to not desire junk food, to not want ice cream, to be happy to turn down the cake, and to not be tempted by the drive-thru, you actually need to love your life. It's vital to be so excited by the person you are, and the direction that you're headed, that you no longer have the appetite for anything that take years from your life. Once you give yourself permission to enjoy the person you naturally are, you will feel compelled to seek the adequate nutrition your body needs to thrive.

If an emotional dependency has manifested as a vicious habit in your life, then it's highly probable that many other aspects of your identity have been morphed by it as well. If you continue to be the same person, with the same behaviours and beliefs, then you will continue to call upon the same emotional triggers to further drive your current personality. You have no choice but to change if you truly want to heal. All you have to do is grant yourself permission to empower your life.

The intention behind your projects (motivation vs. inspiration) has the power to physically take a toll on the body or heal the body. Let me explain.

I really enjoy storytelling, and I just love assembling words. Everyone who knows me could attest to how much I get a thrill out of telling a story. I get really animated and deeply descriptive. So, it makes sense that I've chosen to write. As a result, I feel even more purposeful when I write about the subjects in life I am most inspired by. I am sure it has become quite obvious that my passions lay within the science, health, and arts arenas. Ultimately, I decided to let my heart guide me and I followed its path.

To unite my interests, I began my writing journey many years ago by starting a wellness blog. At the time, my family didn't really like the idea of me being so public, but I felt it was the right choice for me. As soon as I logged onto my website and tapped away at my keyboard, nothing else seemed to matter; time felt like it stopped. I became present and focused, a sense of tranquility filling my mind and calmness sweeping into my space. This is a state where you are focused on nothing more than your creative expression. Some also like to refer to it as being in the zone. It's a blessed place to be.

It is my belief that creativity and healing are very strongly intertwined. The human body has always fascinated me, but I believe I became most enamoured by our design when I was fortunate enough to learn about the direct link between creativity and healing. I'll never forget the day I fully understood this concept. A light bulb went off in my head, and I realized that limiting our creative expression is a detriment to our health.

We have already learned that there are two parts to our autonomic nervous system—our SNS (fight, flight, or freeze) and our PNS (rest and relaxation). We also know that in moments of peril, we switch to SNS. We release stress hormones, two of which are adrenaline and cortisol. Adrenaline (also known as epinephrine), which is excreted by the adrenal glands, creates that great surge of energy. Cortisol, which is also a product of the adrenal glands, is synthesized from cholesterol and is very addictive. It counteracts insulin, contributing to a raise in blood sugar (more fuel for running or battle). Together, these hormones not only heighten our senses, but they also increase our heart rate and send blood away from our vital organs and into our muscles, among many other things. If we perceive the threat to be smaller than us, we fight it, and if we perceive it to be bigger than us, we run from it. Sometimes we deem it's best to just freeze. Hence the term "paralyzed with fear."

During PNS (the state in which our body repairs itself) our digestion takes place, where the immune system becomes active, the reproductive systems kick in, and proper growth takes place. The two nervous systems work independently of each other. In other words, you cannot be in both systems simultaneously. Either you are in perceived jeopardy and your body is in a reactive state, pumped up and prepared for battle, or you are healing. At no stage is your body able to do both at the same time. This is because digestion, immunity, reproduction, growth, and repair are extremely metabolically expensive. Cortisol reduces bone formation, inhibits collagen formation, and slows down wound healing, as well as many other things. Our cleverly designed bodies know that during a threat, these other systems are not critical to our survival, and rather the energy needs to be utilized to run from a tiger, or perhaps a tsunami.

Sure, it's not often we have to run from a tiger these days (thankfully), but we now understand that any perceived threat or stress can kick your body into fight or flight. Constant worry, anxiety, fear of the future, stressful jobs, break-ups, doing tasks we detest, and so on, have the ability to keep our bodies in a perpetual state of fight or flight. Consistent negative stress is not what we have been designed to handle or endure. We are meant to rely on SNS to assist us in a very short brush with danger, not on an ongoing basis. Once we have either outrun the tiger or we somehow managed to kill it with our bare hands, we would then lay under a tree somewhere and relax, or we'd work with a community on some special task.

This continual state of emergency we currently live in means we are not giving our bodies enough time in rest and relaxation. Even when we do sit down to rest, due to our tendency to reflect on events, we may have a hard time turning our mind away from the recent crisis. Thus, we remain in distress. Turning it off just feels so hard, if not impossible.

Okay, so what does this have to do with creativity and healing?

Deep creative expression, or "the zone," if you prefer, is only possible when you are in PNS. This means if you are doing something you love — engaging in something that requires no outside motivation, but simply comes from a place of inspiration, where hours can just pass by and you have completely lost your sense of time and space — then you have forced your brain to switch into a place where you are quite literally healing. This is why you might hear someone claim that playing an instrument feels therapeutic. If it feels like therapy, that is because it actually is!

Writing required me to push through a lot of insecurities, as it puts me at greater risk of being judged, ridiculed, and scrutinized by the world at large. I had a whole list of reasons not to do it. I was someone who used her high school English class as a spare block to hang out with friends more than anything else. It was with great difficulty that I came to the idea that I had any right to choose a life filled with writing.

My family seemed to value skills like math over art. I'd never really known anyone in my immediate circle who had successfully made a career from writing. There were so many motivating reasons why I could have denied myself permission to write. However, once I learned the benefit of abandoning all those worries and just doing what I loved, as it relates to my wellbeing, it became an integral part of my overall wellness routine. It became just as important as exercising, eating well, studying science and nutrition, and meditating.

Being in the zone means you are focused. It implies that you are fully present and mindfully engaged in the task at hand. When something is new, interesting, and challenging, we naturally pay more attention. We feel gripped by it. If you remember from Chapter 9, mindfulness helps increase activity in the left prefrontal cortex (L-PFC), while inhibiting activity of the amygdala (processes emotions) along with the right prefrontal cortex (R-PFC). People with negative moods tend to exhibit heightened activity of the R-PFC and the amygdala. Practicing mindfulness gives you a means of detaching from those negative thoughts that are undoubtedly swirling around. We know that the more you do something, the better at it you become. Our ability to focus works by the same logic. I believe there is no more captivating way to activate the L-PFC than in a fit of creative expression.

It's uncommon for a person to be totally present each and every moment of the day. Nearly everyone drifts in and out of default mode network at some stage. Yet, ruminating over the past and obsessing about the future can negatively impact one's emotional set point. So what is default mode network (DMN) there for? Why do we spend so much time wandering from the present to floating in an imaginary space? If it exists, then it must serve an evolutionary purpose, and it must be to our advantage. It seems that we are designed to reflect and let our imagination get carried away. It looks as though trouble appears when we don't have a goal to work toward.

The less you reflect on a specific project or task, the more free time and space your mind has to fall into a reverie about random, arbitrary things. An absence of a project creates a void that your mind is consequently given liberty to occupy with much less productive things. In other words, if it's not given a challenge to overcome, it goes and finds one. The mind needs to be pushed to new heights and greater complexity or it is at risk of becoming unstimulated. It longs for a puzzle to work through. Your body is your mind's servant, but your mind is the subordinate to your heart. When your mind is forced to surrender its will to the will of your heart, you begin to live an inspired life.

Pattern Recognition

In cognitive neuroscience and psychology, the term *pattern recognition* is used to label a cognitive process that matches data from a stimulus with data retrieved from memory. Some of the ways in which we recognize patterns are through units of music, language, physical features, symbols, and a variety of other things. Pattern recognition happens automatically, although it doesn't always happen instantly. Nonetheless, pattern recognition is an innate ability that is common to all animals. It represents a deep instinct to establish order of the world. We have the innate drive to organise chaos so that we can impose rules and order, thus ensuring our world becomes more survivable.

You can imagine how useful this tool would have been to our ancestors, and still is for us today. Our ability to recognize patterns helps us discern between the facial features of our loved ones and that of a tiger lurking in the distance. We have applied this skill in the invention of tools. After our ancestors began to walk upright, we were able to use our hands to pick things up and create instruments to better our chances at survival. The most useful of tools became popular, and traditions were formed based on what patterns were revealed to have worked the best.

At the time of this writing, humans are thought to be the world's best pattern-producing machines. Our brains possess unique features including intelligence, language, imagination, invention, and belief in the imaginary. We have some advantage over our four-legged friends; being upright exposes us to new sensory information. Our ears can draw input from an expanded audio space, and our eyes are exposed to a greater field of vision. Four-legged animals are limited to a rather confined field of vision and other sensory information. The capacity to accurately detect a pattern is limited to the sphere of awareness. If it weren't for our ability to travel to and capture detailed images of the moon, it would be easy to mistake the rock formations on its surface for some mystical face. Space technology has allowed us to raise our level of awareness so we can have a more precise explanation for the face that appears on the moon.

Our brain just loves a good riddle. In fact, if it finds no familiar pattern, it attempts to make one up. The more diffused the stimulus, the easier we could mistake it for some other thing. *Apophenia* describes the tendency to see patterns that do not actually exist, and we all share in exhibiting this trait. An example of apophenia would include our knack to find faces or figures in clouds. Another illustration would be that we often link causal relationships between events that are, in fact, unrelated.

Much of the confidence we have about ourselves, and our respective lives, for that matter, is based on conclusions that are drawn from patterns we believe we have recognized. However, our beliefs can become victim to our limited understanding of the big picture, and thus, so can our opinions of ourselves. Your ability to recognize where you display the traits of a genius is confined to the borders of your experience. It makes sense, then, that the more you apply yourself to challenges that lift you to new heights, the more opportunities you will have to raise your level of awareness, and thus recognize much more precise patterns in your life.

You may feel compelled to say that you are not creative and do not have the ability to heal through creative expression. But I am here to reiterate that that is simply not true; we are all creative beings. Any activity that you can get lost in—cooking, painting, gardening, etc.— are all spaces where you are healing. We tend to equate creativity only to the arts, but to create is to simply bring something new into the world. That newness can be anything—a solution to a problem, a product, a service, a game, or even an experience. The choice is truly our own to discover and to bring forth. If something piques your interest, captures your attention and challenges you to greater complexity, why wouldn't you give yourself permission to do it?

People just love to attest that they don't know what they came here to do. They look me dead in the eye and claim that they are lost. "Yes you do! Everyone knows what inspires them," I say. They shake their head and stick to their respective case. "What would you do if you had all the money in the world, and you couldn't fail?" I ask. "If you didn't fear the opinions of those that matter the most to you? If you believed that you were smart enough, strong enough, and beautiful enough? If you didn't fear that you were going against the ideals of some religious authority?"

Without fail, they smirk. "Well in that case, I would..." they reply.

"So you do know what you want to do, you've just reasoned your way out," I explain.

When we make other people our authority, we let their opinions take primary influence over our lives. For example, when an idea has struck, we then spend countless hours weighing the risks or rewards. The thought that someone won't like it shakes us to our very core. It evokes such anxiety within us that we become paralyzed by it. It doesn't matter what you do, someone won't care much for it.

Sturt Hinton, founder of Frequency H2O, had a vision. In 2012, he quit his high-paying job because he no longer found it fulfilling. He spent a year in the small town of Noosa, Australia, where he reflected upon his life. He had no idea what he would do next, and his money was quickly running dry. He shared with some friends and family that he had an idea that he felt called to create. He explained that he wanted to offer the world a new type of water. He wanted to energize it with the frequency of love. They all said he had gone mad.

He made his way to Townsville, Australia, because he learned that Townsville was a premium source of spring water. It was there that he got 20 bottles of his unique idea made up. He spent his last $300 on a plane ticket to Sydney and he stuffed his backpack with the 20 litres of love. With barely enough pocket change to make bus fare, he put on his backpack and made his way to all the health shops in Sydney that he could find. With nothing but a dream and 20 bottles of water, he walked into store after store. When he got to the first store, the buyer heard his pitch and said, "That is the stupidest idea I have ever heard," and Sturt was laughed out.

Sturt happens to be a dear friend of mine. We met each other about a week after he arrived in Sydney. I was the buyer at a health store at the time. On the day we first met, there was a terrible storm. Sturt walked through the doors of the shop I was working at, and he was soaked from head to toe. Now, he's a very handsome man, but the moment I met him, he looked more like a drowned rat. "I love it," I said, after he gave me his speech. Of course, I was a bit sceptical whether the customers would buy it, but I gave it a chance, and so did a few other stores. At first he would drop off the deliveries himself, and we took a liking to each other and became friends.

The water spread like wildfire! It took Sydney by storm. Within mere months, he was in hundreds of stores. After a year he went national, and before he reached two years, his water went global. Every single day he'd heard, "No." He had no idea what he was doing. He just took it one day at a time. With one step in front of the other, he changed his whole life. He brought something new into the world that made people happy. Some people hate it, and some people love it. That's life.

We don't have the ability to accurately foretell future events. It's a futile way to expend our energy. What we do have reign over, however, is our own body, so bring the focus back inside and redirect your energy towards the act of personal healing. Whatever belief you hold that limits you from doing something that inspires you, it's time to retire it, as those limiting beliefs are literally killing you.

My desire is for you to blow your own mind and expand your limits. To fuel your projects with empowering emotions instead of disempowering states that only produce weeds. To engage in a life that actually interests you, that grabs your attention, and moves you to exercise your talents. With enough repetition and focus, you have the ability to master anything you desire. The only way you'll want to show up day after day and apply yourself is to do things that are meaningful to you. Listen to the demands of your heart while you hold faith in its interests—despite the dialogue with your anxieties. Eventually, with enough practice, you will be better able to distinguish between the two, and the only reward you will be addicted to is personal gratification.

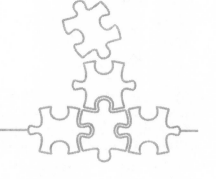

CHAPTER 13

Cultivation

P racticing mindfulness while being in the embrace of a project that you love is all well and good, if you have an adequate amount of time and space to dedicate to your mission. Sometimes taking steps towards a fully inspired life can be a bit of a long transition. What if you don't currently have the freedom to detach from negative emotions by diving head first into your passion projects at any hour of the day? It might be frowned upon if you told your boss that you're stressed-out, and you'd like to take the day off to go paint (unless, of course, they employ you as a painter). Sure, you can find the time before or after work, or perhaps on your weekends, but it's not realistic for us to turn our backs on all our responsibilities. How, then, can you turn the stress response off in the moments when you can't do the waltz with your creative mission?

To prune out old thinking, we need something to be able to turn our attention away from those unsightly thoughts. It's fairly easy to acknowledge when your mind is being swept by your negative emotions, but it's not so easy to stop it. In the moments when we get caught ruminating over frightening past and present scenarios, we require something that's always available and sustainable to turn to. Exercising reason usually doesn't stop the stress response, because the amygdala (in a more primitive and reactive part of our brain) is often the site that provokes the stress response, and the amygdala doesn't respond to reasoning. Reasoning, rather, is a function of cortex-based processing. Think of it as though it has overheated; something needs to be able to instantly and effectively cool it off.

There are easy, free, and always accessible tools we can use to turn our fight-or-flight response off relatively quickly, which will simultaneously switch us over to rest and relaxation. Some people will find that one of the methods listed below will work more effectively than others, and some will find that using a combination of two or more of these tools is the best approach that works for them. With a little bit of practice, you will be able to determine which is most influential for you.

Relaxation techniques are generally considered safe for healthy people, although some report increased anxiety with specific techniques, while they find others extremely helpful. As with anything, it is paramount that you find what works best for you given your current circumstances. People with serious physical or mental health problems should discuss relaxation techniques with their healthcare providers. None of these techniques provided are meant to be a viable substitute for professional therapy, nor are they listed with the intention of providing a cure for any mental or physical disease. So, if you believe you may suffer from a mental disorder, consult with a medical professional immediately.

Diaphragmatic Breathing

Also known as abdominal breathing, diaphragmatic breathing is among the most effective ways to turn off SNS while activating PNS. Yogis refer to it as pranic breathing. By modulating the breath you narrow the focus, bringing yourself back into the present moment, and it further relaxes the body by massaging the internal organs. Diaphragmatic breathing slows down the heart rate, allows for increased oxygen flow through the body, and helps the muscles relax, which all turn off the stress response. Most people feel an almost instant shift in their physiology when they engage in diaphragmatic breathing.

In the beginning, this way of breathing may feel a bit strange, but soon you will become familiar with the technique. You should be able to reduce stress in a matter of moments by taking a few deep breaths. When you breathe from your abdomen (or diaphragm), your belly will expand and move out with each inhalation. Your chest will rise ever so slightly, but a great deal of the movement will be from your abdomen. The inhale breath should be long and steady, followed by the exhale breath that you can allow to occur naturally.

Muscle Relaxation Techniques

Progressive muscle relaxation (PMR) is a form of stress management that was first developed by American physician Edmund Jacobson. PMR is a systematic technique in which the subject is trained to voluntarily relax individual muscles. Jacobson's method involved the tensing and relaxation of 16 muscle groups. The stress response leads to muscle tension, so this method of intentionally relaxing the muscles encourages a relaxed state by reducing central nervous system activity. In 1984, Joseph Wolpe established a method called abbreviated progressive relaxation training (APRT), which focuses on relaxing several muscle groups simultaneously.

In the current day, the art of relaxation therapy takes on many different forms, as several therapists have developed various methods of muscle relaxation techniques over the years.

You will want to find a place where you will not be interrupted, as a full session of muscle relaxation should take about 10 to 15 minutes. Progressive relaxation can be done standing, sitting, or lying down, but some find they fall asleep if it's performed lying down.

Once in position, close your eyes, uncross your legs, and let your hands rest comfortably at your sides or on your lap. As soon as you have found a comfortable position, let your eyes close. Take a deep and steady breath in through the nostrils. Let the abdomen expand on the inhale, and allow yourself to relax as you exhale. After a few deep breaths, you can begin muscle relaxation. Tensing is done as you inhale, then relax and release all the tension as you exhale. Slowly and deliberately work one muscle group at a time. Be careful not to rush; take your time between each step. Allow each muscle group to feel completely loose and limp before proceeding to the next group. Some prefer to start at the feet and others choose to begin by tensing and relaxing the facial muscles.

Single Focus

Single Focus is just as it sounds — where the object being focused upon is held in the mind without consciousness wavering from it. The point of concentration can be whatever the individual chooses, but it is thought to be most effective when focused on the breath. The Sanskrit translation for "single focus" or "holding steady" is known as *dharana*. If your gaze is the single point of focus, it is known as a *drishti*. Holding steady in one point of concentration keeps the mind from floating off into DMN, and helps us detach from our mind chatter. Concentrating on a single point of focus is an instant and effective way of practicing mindfulness that steers the mind away from the past or future, right into the present moment. Many find it to be an increased benefit to focus on both the breath and either a visual point of focus or a specific word.

Focusing on a single word (also known as a mantra) while bringing attention to the breath helps condition the mind, so that in the future the word will help trigger relaxation. If you have chosen to use a mantra, it is best if the word (or words) have a significant meaning. It could be symbolic of relaxation, a shift, or cultivating change. Examples are *new*, *change*, *now*, *peace*, or *switch*. Om shanti is among the most popular mantras. *Om* is thought to be the sound of the universe, and *shanti* means peace, rest, calmness, tranquillity, or bliss. Using a mantra with two syllables makes it easier to connect it with the breath, as you focus on one syllable during the in breath, and the second syllable is in conjunction with the out breath.

Metacognition

Although not considered a relaxation tool, meta-cognition is an excellent tool that can be useful when forming new habits. Tune in often, and let your awareness acknowledge all the various pathways a negative emotion takes to drive your actions, behaviours, and habits. Awareness will help you quickly recognize the next time you act out one of its traits. The sooner you catch it and stop it in its tracks, the more effective the synaptic pruning process will be.

Insight is useless without change, so take action and do it immediately. It's fundamental to stop the behaviours that are sourced from the old emotions the moment you acknowledge that you're acting them out, and then swiftly replace that behaviour with a new process that works towards the goals in your life you want to create.

Identify your most commonly used weapon. When I refer to weapons, I am referring to the SNS response you most often play out in a moment of duress. Do you tend to resort to flight (fleeing stressful situations), fight (becoming aggressive), or freeze (becoming paralyzed)? We all have the inclination to respond to specific stressors with a particular weapon. The stressor is simply a trigger that signals the autonomic nervous system to react in a particular way. Sometimes, we can use a combination of weapons, but being creatures of habit, we typically tend to favour one set of armour in similar situations, and we may use another weapon for an entirely different scenario altogether.

For example, you may find you tend to freeze during a social conflict, but you lean towards fight in business conflicts. Bringing light to which weapon you are more inclined to use in a specific setting helps your conscious mind identify when you are actually using your weapon and acting with the intention of surviving rather than thriving.

Surviving means you are trying. You may remember in an earlier chapter I described trying as the antithesis of being. If you are operating from the SNS perspective, then it is because you are resisting something, or there is a force of some kind that you are pushing against. Now, if there is no real and present danger in the immediate environment, and thought alone has triggered the need to draw a weapon, it is that very thought that you are resisting. There is nothing from the outside world that requires you to draw your weapon, so to speak.

It stands to reason then that the beliefs and emotions underlying that thought reveal the source of the force that you are pushing against. These uncomfortable feelings are an insight into what beliefs about yourself and your life may be creating cognitive dissonance, and thus cause you to subconsciously sabotage your goals. Until one's beliefs are in alignment and behaviours are in accordance with a desire, they are not yet in the necessary state of being that is required to obtain that goal.

After careful investigation, you will find that the belief that most often leads to cognitive dissonance is the main limiting belief that runs your life and determines whether or not you successfully obtain each of your goals. Each of us can have many hindering beliefs that create an internal struggle. We are not limited to being conditioned solely by one belief. You may find, however, that one belief emerges more often than others, and its consistent negative narrative impacts the success of many of your goals. Because the belief, or thoughts about that belief, can generate a specific negative emotion, the redundancy of that thought is likely to have led to an emotional dependency.

At first it may be hard to determine which emotions dominate your thoughts, but there is a way to assess them. When your mind wanders into DMN, you have indeed become lost in thought. I like to divide these wandering thoughts into three categories: nightmares (or daymares), fantasies, and dreams.

Nightmares/Daymares (negatively charged)

Our natural emotional set point (as long as we aren't in present danger) should reflect joy and peace. If you are lost in nightmares, you are dialoguing about or working through a future problem that you are convincing yourself you'll run into, or you are dwelling about something you feel resentful about in the past. Therefore, if you are lost in these types of thoughts, you aren't feeling peaceful. You are clearly being consumed by some negative emotion. I refer to those types of thoughts as nightmares. They are not always deeply terrifying, as there are different degrees of nightmares (or daymares, if that's what you prefer to call them).

Once you have identified that you are having a waking nightmare, try and avoid the need to judge it. Judging your thoughts just produces more of the same negative feelings and emotions. Remember that the amygdala (which processes emotions) does not respond to reasoning, so that form of analysis is not conducive to a quick physiological change. What you can do is use the innate ability awarded to us all—metacognition— to let your mind take notice of the behaviour. Soon you will be able to notice patterns and commonalities between your haunting thoughts; at which point, if you choose, you can use the method that I have named "The Three B's," which is an easy and effective three-step process that I've listed in subsequent paragraphs. These steps can be used in order to change unwanted thinking patterns while cultivating new ones.

Fantasies (positively charged)

If you are envisioning some future event that implies a "happily ever after," you are not operating from peace. You are attached to an outcome, and expecting something that doesn't exist. You are still viewing the world through an elevated emotional goggle; instead of the emotion being a negative one, the fantasy creates a positively charged emotion. Despite the fact that it feels good, if it's not truthful and obtainable, it can be toxic. Eventually, when life doesn't live up to the fantasy of happily ever after, we feel as though we have failed at life. But we didn't actually fail. We simply aimed for a goal that is unobtainable and unrealistic instead of striving for goals that inspire us. These are neither useful nor truthful thoughts and beliefs. The notion that something could potentially get in the way of these fantasies can quickly activate the stress response.

Dreams

These are new ideas, productive dialogue, wild imaginations, and purposeful thoughts that you are having, and they relate to the things you want to create. They don't all have to be correlated to one specific thing you want to create; you can design several things at once. These types of thoughts are productive; they help you expand towards your missions, and they are from a peaceful state. Your physiology in the moments when you are lost in these types of thoughts will feel like a reflection of that peaceful and joyful state.

As soon as your conscious mind acknowledges that you have been led astray by nightmares, you can use the simple and effective Three B's Method.

Step 1. Breathe

(Use the PNS activating tools listed previously.) Choose the one (or more) that proves to work the most efficiently to detach your focus from the thoughts (diaphragmatic breathing; dharana; muscle relaxation or body scan, etc.). Shifting your focus to your breath and away from the unwanted thoughts is like cutting off the emotion's umbilical cord. Over time, with the absence of your attention, it will starve to death.

Step 2. Believe

Once the stress response has been turned off and you feel relaxed and focused on the present moment, assess the limiting belief that has triggered you to get caught in old lines of thinking. Then bring to mind the new beliefs that you would rather subscribe to instead.

Step 3. Behave

Cultivate change by finally steering your thoughts in a new direction that is in alignment with your goals, and perform a new routine or behaviour that leads to satisfying rewards, such as your new goals.

Your attention on these thoughts keeps the emotion alive, and your behaviours that result from it feed it, so it's important to follow through with all of these steps if you want to create a real change.

Fantasies are not as innocuous as we would like to believe. Fantasies and nightmares often come in pairs (as do cravings and aversions), and it's for this reason that fantasies should be treated the same way as nightmares, and it's as if you have to retrain your brain at all hours of the day, which can be exhausting and frustrating. The old emotions, thoughts, and beliefs will keep resurfacing—especially in the early stages of reconditioning—but persistence is the key. It may feel as though you are training a very wild animal, but there will be a point in which that animal suddenly begins to surrender. This is in part due to the forgetting curve.

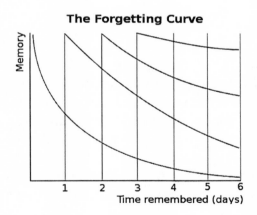

Figure 1.

The forgetting curve, shown in Figure 1, was first published in the late 1880s by psychologist Hermann Ebbinghaus, and it shows how information is lost over time when there is no attempt to retain it. The forgetting curve purports to show that we have the tendency to halve the retention of newly learned material within a matter of days unless the information is intentionally retained. Hence the phrase, "Use it or lose it."

As you can see from the figure, the early stage of new learning—and thus the initial stage breaking an old habit while memorizing a new one—is the most fragile stage. If you quit before the wild animal quits, then you are training it to be even more defiant. Stick with it, even when it seems pointless. We hold the belief that we can train a dog to sit if we have enough persistence, so we just repeatedly attempt to train them until they learn. Training your subconscious works exactly the same way. You just have to hold faith and be relentless in your pursuit. Eventually you will, just all of a sudden, find yourself in new unconscious patterns.

Meditation

Many find the word *meditation* unpalatable because of its association with mysticism. Meditation called me for ages. Every time I heard the word, it piqued my interest. Something inside told me to investigate it, but I didn't invite it into my life due to my limited beliefs about what it represented. I find the mystical world to be highly intriguing, but I am a girl who devours science and proven facts. You can imagine my absolute elation as I discovered that the two were, in fact, united. Nothing tickles me more than when old spiritual teachings and new scientific findings merge.

The subconscious mind processes a great deal more information than our conscious mind has the ability to. If we close our eyes, we cut off a huge portion of the sensory information the mind has to process. Sitting in a quiet room with earplugs, or wearing earphones with relaxing music playing, mutes the distracting auditory signals coming from the external world. At this stage, we are able to draw our senses inward, and the internal world becomes the primary focus, making it more real than anything else.

Using the relaxation tools previously listed, combined with a single point of focus, enables us to detach from our analytical thoughts while simultaneously slipping into a deeply relaxed state. The single point of focus will ultimately lead the analytical mind to let go, or to at least turn down its volume. In this place, the mind chatter slows down. For experienced meditators, there can be gaps absent of any thought at all—although this does take some practice.

Once the mind is calm and the thoughts have slowed down, they are easier to observe as they float in. The meditator can allow a thought to come in; through metacognition, they can acknowledge the thought and then choose to let it fade away. Another thought can come in, and it too can fade away. What better way to become familiar with the automatic thoughts that just fire off at will inside your mind? It's a beautiful experience to be able to acknowledge a thought without judgement and then make the choice to just let it go. This tradition not only gives us a means to better know ourselves, but also devotes us to a practice that is dedicated to detaching from, and further controlling, our thoughts—which is a skill that, like any other skill, can be strengthened over time.

The Tibetan word for meditation is *gom,* which means "to become familiar with." The English word *meditation* is derived from the Latin verb *meditari,* meaning "to think, contemplate, devise, ponder." As impressive as this all sounds, there is something more about this practice that might blow your mind.

Meditation opens the gate between the conscious and subconscious mind; it can act as a means to get into the shed where the gardener of your life keeps its blueprints, its instructions, and many of its secrets. We meditate because the subconscious is highly prone to suggestibility in this state, just as we are during the process of hypnosis. One of the main purposes of self-hypnosis (another word for meditation) is to go beyond the conscious mind so we can change unwanted beliefs, behaviours, emotional reactions, and various unconscious states of being. Further, it's a tool to recover many of our motives that are unknown to our conscious mind.

When we are awake and alert in normal consciousness, we are operating in what is known as Beta consciousness. Beta brainwave cycles are between 13 to about 30 cycles per second. In highly stressful or aroused states, we can go into high Beta brainwave patterns. In Beta, we are very aware of our body, the environment, and time. A sense of immediate urgency and the tendency to think selfishly is a dead giveaway that you are in a high Beta brainwave pattern.

Once a meditator disconnects from the distractions in the external environment, transcends the feelings in the body, and allows themselves to lose track of time and space, they can move from Beta brainwave patterns to Alpha, or even down to Theta. We slip in and out of Alpha state naturally in the moments when we first awaken in the morning and just as we are falling asleep at night.

When the pineal gland stops producing melatonin (the hormone that makes you fall asleep) and instead serotonin is produced, or vice versa, we are in this trance-like state known as Alpha. During moments of deep creative thinking we can also drift into this state. Alpha cycles are about 8 to 13 cycles per second, when measured by an electroencephalograph (EEG).

The Theta brainwave state, just below Alpha, is the desired meditative state. Initially it may take some practice to reach Theta without drifting off into deep sleep, which produces a Delta brainwave pattern. Our mind is highly suggestible in Alpha and Theta states because the volume to the analytical mind has been turned down. In these lower brainwaves we can recondition the subconscious mind by uniting vivid imaginations and feelings. We can intentionally rehearse future potential outcomes by envisioning them, and then allow ourselves to feel as though that outcome has already occurred. We reflect on previous experiences with a new lens and generate new emotions associated with those memories. Through repetition we can go from a state of thinking about, and thus trying to be, a new person with new beliefs and a transformed personal reality to truly being that person.

In Theta, it is as though your body is asleep but your mind is awake. In this state you're at liberty to imagine, to create, and to change the unconscious patterns without the judgement of the analytical mind. Children—whom you will find are highly suggestible—are functioning in the Theta brainwave between the ages of about 2 and 5 years old. As they reach the ages between 5 and 8, their brain begins to demonstrate higher patterns (in the Alpha state), at which point the analytical mind starts to develop. We have come to understand that children start to establish set beliefs and laws about the world during these years. As a result, their level of suggestibility declines.

To meditate is to become familiar with one's true self and choices. Creative visualisation is effective when we are peaceful and open. By thinking in detail of the picture we have in our mind's eye of a healed life, we can actually begin to simultaneously feel those emotions as if we had lived the experience. This process allows your mind and body to experience the outcome before it's manifested in the external environment.

Through reflecting on the self—past, present, and future—we can contemplate events in a deeply relaxed state. Often it is in this space where we recognize how a series of synchronises have brought us where we are now in the present, allowing us to be more grateful for all the experiences in our past.

Many believe that they can't meditate, and speak of it as if it's a power that only a few possess. They claim that they have made attempts, but they just couldn't do it. If you are one of those individuals who has bought into this belief, let me remind you that you did not know how to walk until you learned how to do that, either. Meditation is a practice, and a skill we develop. Just like any other practice, it takes some time and effort, but it is available and extremely beneficial to all.

There are different meditation types, such as creative meditation, guided meditation, astral, prayer, or reflective, and what is known as still mind meditation. In still mind meditation there is no time or attachments. To learn more about meditation as a practice you can refer to my website, www.mariaayne.com. Here you can also find the program "The Eating Enigma: 90 days to transforming your relationship with food," which includes a series of meditations that work through emotional dependencies, limiting beliefs, and unhealthy behaviours in a systematic approach. You also have access to a variety of other methods that best suit you, as there are a vast selection of guided meditations available online. Or you can practice meditation on your own daily.

Initially the mind will wander, and the moments where your mind feels clear may be brief. But with time and practice (just like everyone else who works at it), you will be able to quiet the mind for just as much time as you need to be able to observe the thoughts. With dedication and repetition, your ability to meditate will increase.

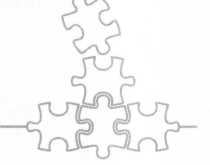

CHAPTER 14

Disclosure

Disclose who you no longer want to be

You have now gained a greater understanding of how holding onto an emotion gives the emotion the power to control your life, your thoughts, and your attention, while driving your overall behaviour. Every moment of your life will be subject to distortion through that emotional lens. Remember that it is our thoughts that have the ability to create emotion, but it is our emotions that also have the ability to drive our thoughts; they focus our attention and filter our reality. In essence, we get more of the same thing that we put out.

Your perception of a past event, and the emotions associated with that event, have branded you. It has filled your garden with a weed that must be eradicated if you want your new flowers to bloom. Nothing will change until we allow ourselves to look back on the past through an alternate lens.

For example, if your perception about a past experience makes you feel unworthy, and the emotional charge of that event is strong, you will continue to view life through the lens of unworthiness. You will filter the world to see more of the same thing—further compounding and verifying your unworthiness. With enough repetition, it then becomes a strong belief about yourself and your life, based on evidence that you have collected over time. Proof of your worthiness has always been there, too; it was just never granted access into the gates to your garden (otherwise known as your attention).

The antidote to any emotional charge is the opposite emotion. This means an equal amount of evidence that fully proves your worthiness can, in fact, dissipate the feelings of unworthiness. But what is most challenging is that it is those pesky unworthy feelings that direct your attention, thus hindering you from witnessing your worthiness. The antidote is within your grasp, but your current perception of the event will block your ability to see it.

Now, we know that the events that brand us are the ones we have the greatest emotional charges on. So it stands to reason that other events that don't carry the same amplitude of emotion will have much less power to change our emotional set point, even if the other experiences carry the antidote to the prior experience. Unless the two charges are equal, one will not be able to neutralize the other.

Shifting your perception on that crucial life event and viewing it from a higher understanding is one of the most effective ways to prune the weed. When we spend years being resentful because of some past story, we can recall the drawbacks to our life and see it as doing more harm to us than good. We have a harder time giving the event credit for all the gifts we have also received as a direct result of it.

We become addicted to seeing ourselves as a victim of that story, where some injustice has been inflicted upon us. We refuse to admit that it turned out to be of great service to us in many ways as well. We believe (and really fear) that turning in our resentments and exchanging them for gratitude for the experience means that we are somehow condoning what happened to us. And that simply isn't true.

We have a story, a perception, and a perspective about an event or many events, which bundled together makes up our respective identities—one that we have become dependent on. Who would we be if not for this tale? We'd be stepping into the unknown, and the unknown frightens us. We would be forced to change, to shed an old skin, which exposes us. We would have to take control over our emotions and our life, and thus become the master of our destiny. We would have to take some responsibility for how we feel. We fear that we will lose some of the payoffs that come with this belief, such as support or attention from others. We would often rather stay stuck in a mistruth than transcend the emotion because we are more comfortable with the lie over self-empowerment. We certainly aren't going to let a few facts about how things actually unfolded, and the blessings that have blossomed because of the event, get in the way of continuing to be the only person we know how to be.

Remember, the strong desire to remain a victim to life's circumstances and the addiction to the emotions associated with that narrative are disempowering. They inhibit us from giving ourselves permission to rewrite a new destiny.

190

Give up the story! Resentment is toxic, and creates a deficiency of love and appreciation. If you can't abandon the belief that you were a victim of some misfortune, then you are subscribing to a vicious lie. Is it possible to admit that as tragic as the event may have been at the time of occurrence, the outcome of that story has since proved itself to be quite fortunate in many other respects, and will likely continue to? When you let go of the narrative of victimhood by neutralizing your perception of the event, you dissipate the emotion. You become unhinged from the events of your past.

All of the great leaders to date have been faced with some adversity. Drawing wisdom from their experiences and showing others the way are the key attributes that make them such profound and inspirational leaders. It is not what has happened to you that defines you; it's what you believe about it that counts. The meaning that we assign to these events controls the fate of our lives.

Many will discount the significance of this information. They will dismiss it and claim that it's too easy to be true. Perhaps they will skim through it while claiming that it's nothing they haven't already heard before. This narrative is the old self, desperately attempting to preserve its identity and refusing to step into the unknown. If you have rejected these concepts and labeled them as too good to be true, or maybe you feel that it's too obvious or just too easy, rest assured that it is none of those things.

Breaking an emotional addiction was hands down the hardest—and most rewarding—goal that I have ever committed myself to. Rewiring my brain by pruning out old connections and simultaneously wiring new circuitry was met with resistance at every single step of the way. My garden was riddled with weeds that I had to dedicate enormous amounts of time, energy, and focus to remove. Day after day, I had to use my awareness at all times to determine if I was behaving as my old self or my new self. I had to use this awareness to catch myself in the midst of old behaviour and stop it while choosing a new, unfamiliar route. All of this, without ever really knowing any other reality to be true. I had to hold faith that with enough consistency, I could change my way of being. I had to take responsibility for my life, and I absolutely had to give up the excuses I used as crutches for decades. There was nothing easy about any of that.

There is no room in your new life for both a story of victimhood and a tale of heroism. The two stories can't share the same bed. The stronger of the two states will cancel the other one out.

When you think about it, in order to build anything new, there must be some form of destruction. When we digest food, we have to first break it down before our body can use it to build our tissues. The same logic can be applied to the mind. The old self-deprecating thoughts cannot be left to survive if we want the new, empowered self to have any fighting chance.

Disclose to yourself who you have been and what you no longer want to believe about your life. Make note of your old patterns, and ask yourself the necessary questions to assess the difference between the old you and the new you: How did that limited version of me talk? What did I obsess about? How did that person act? Whom did I surround myself with, and what kind of people would I like to emulate? What trigger foods will I no longer tempt myself with? What new routines will follow environmental triggers? What old payoffs are no longer classified as payoffs, and what are the new rewards I would like to seek? What excuses does the old personality use? What is the payoff of being this old personality?

Recognizing the payoffs of your old patterns is essential because it reveals a strategy by which we get our deep-seated needs met. For example, it's often very difficult for someone to let go of the notion that they are a victim of an experience, because feeling like a victim has rewarded them with attention from those that surround them. Knowing what the payoffs are allows you to consciously make sure those deep-seated needs are continued to be met by alternate means. It's important to keep in mind that cues and rewards don't change when we break a habit; it is the route we take to earn the payoff (the pattern) that can be transformed.

<u>Disclose who you truly are</u>

It's imperative to question every single one of your actions and ask yourself, "Why am I doing this?" Investigate the purpose behind each step you take. Are you doing an action or inaction because of an outside influencer, or are you making this move for your higher self? What thoughts stir up impulsive behaviours? Is it for the greater good of the person you want to become, or is it just a habit from the old personality? Would the person you want to be make the decision to eat this cake? Would the person you want to be react the same way to this situation? Become familiar with the traits from the old emotions that reveal themselves in your actions.

Remember, all good things take time, and there will be moments you feel stuck, or as though your progress has plateaued. This is all part of the journey. We live in a time when instant gratification is available at every turn. When the mood strikes and we can't be bothered to leave our homes, we can simply jump online, order essentially anything, and it can be delivered to our door. If we need a date, we can download an application to our phones and be chatting with a new potential love interest in seconds. Movies, clothes, electronics, cars, you name it—all available with the click of a button. Real personal growth, spiritual development, and mental expansion—these are precious, and they take time and dedication to fully obtain.

It's said that it takes 10,000 hours of dedicated practice to be considered an expert in a field, but in today's world, everyone wants to be successful overnight. It takes a lifetime to acquire real wisdom, and yet many hold the expectation that a few books are all you need. Remember that the goals that matter, the goals that you are inspired to achieve, are nothing like the things you can obtain by shopping online. They are a way of life; they are a practice. These goals require dedication to a cause—your cause—and they won't give you instant gratification. But they will be even better because if you keep at it, you'll get steady doses of personal gratification, and that's even more priceless. Never give up; it really is about the journey. Be careful not to have unrealistic expectations about yourself, life, and time, because an unmet unrealistic expectation sets us up for failure. When committing to a change, you have to completely embody the change before your universe shifts around you, and that will take patience and dedication.

Keystone habits, as Charles Duhigg describes in the book, *The Power of Habit*, are good habits that indirectly lead to other good habits. Some of these would include writing down your daily goals, eating well, meditating, or exercising daily. These habits have a substantial effect on both our mental and emotional health, and consequently affect every other area of our life.

When setting out a new goal, it is imperative to determine what keystone habits the type of person who obtains said goal engages in daily. Ask yourself: "What action steps can I realistically take each day?" and, "What new rituals do I need to implement in order find myself in a new paradigm, and ultimately a new reality where I am truly comfortable with being me?" Write down your responses; you will be thoroughly amazed that you already possess the knowledge you need to obtain your goal.

Remember, the most important thing in your wellness journey is to be authentic to your true nature. It is paramount for you to be sincere to your own personal values—by releasing negatively imposed ideas of who you think you should be, what you should believe, and what other people think you should be doing, and focusing instead on celebrating your own unique desires and gifts. Trust that you will find the most inspiring way to share these gifts with the rest of humanity. I assure you, if an inspiring goal is highly valuable to you, then it's highly valuable to many others, and that means the world needs you.

My disclosure

I need to disclose a secret. This book was written for me. For the little girl inside who had a holy communion with nothing but ice cream, devised for the young woman with so many questions and a hopeless realization that no one was coming to save her with their answers. The desire to write this book has been my greatest desire for the lion's share of my life. The ability to get there—to take action towards every single moment that made this book become a reality—was governed solely by my faith. To me, it was a direct measure of how much my chosen beliefs either limited me or freed me.

The concept for this book was once just an itty-bitty seed, crying out for its cord to a life force energy, secretly shrouded under the leaves of doubt and worry. For years, I whispered to myself quietly inside that it would be really nice if one day I could be the person who writes this story. And for several years after softly saying these words, I started to entertain the notion that, just maybe, I could.

Over time, I continually chose to understand and embrace the concept that I could make my dream a reality. My secret garden could be filled with flowers of inspiration and trees of fulfilment if I simply committed, moment after moment, day after day, to have faith in my little secret garden. It was then that I was able to open the gates, where from the inside I had all the resources I needed to endure all the planting and pruning, and any-thing else necessary to make it happen. To learn enough, apply myself enough, work hard enough towards the goal that truly served me along with humanity. I contin-ually nurtured that seed and gave myself the blessing to obtain something that, at one time, I felt too ashamed to even dare declare I wanted.

And, just like that, nothing else mattered more. There was no vacant room available in my focus for anything but my new goal—certainly no spare occupancy for thoughts of what I didn't want. There was no free time to waste on old compulsions; my greater goals took an unprecedented priority. As my secret garden bloomed, so did my admiration for it, which eradicated any tolerance for an infestation of weeds. Lies, limiting beliefs, and urges no longer possessed me.

So there you go. Do the work, plant your seeds, give them life force energy, nurture them, give them plush soil to live in, tend to your secret garden, and eventually, with faith, you can be free.

Okay… maybe it is a bit of a how-to guide.

Thank you for visiting my secret garden. May it inspire you to tend more lovingly to yours, so we can come together as a species and form one little magical universal field filled with love, compassion, and creativity.

For more information on how you can apply these tools to cultivate a long-lasting and meaningful change, visit www.mariaayne.com.

Acknowledgements

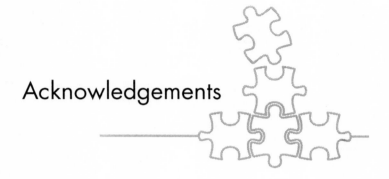

A very special thank you goes to my extraordinary friend Lora Liao, who advised me through every step in the process of writing this book. Also to my dear friends Cara Meehan and Patrick Trivuncevic, who supported me in every way possible. I could not imagine having gone through this process without the three of you. I am forever grateful.

While there are too many names to identify individually, I want to extend my gratitude to all of my family, friends, colleagues, and even to the strangers who encouraged me and contributed their insights throughout this past year. This book would not be the same without your contributions, so thank you.

Bibliography

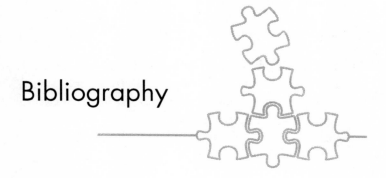

Adams, O. Peter. 2013. "The Impact of Brief High-Intensity Exercise on Blood Glucose Levels." *Diabetes, Metabolic Syndrome and Obesity: Targets and Therapy* 6: 113-122. Accessed Jun 12, 2017.

Alexander, Bruce K. 2001. "The Myth of Drug-Induced Addiction." *Canadian Senate*. Accessed Dec 12, 2004. http://www.parl.gc.ca/37/1/parlbus/commbus/senate/com-e/ille-e/presentation-e/alexender-e.htm.

2017. "Alpha Wave." *Wikipedia*. Jun 17. Accessed Jul 6, 2017.

Altenmuller, E. 2003. "Focal Dystonia: Advances in Brain Imaging and Understanding of Fine Motor Control in Musicians." *Hand Clin* 19: 1-16.

Arden, J. B. 2014. *The Brain Bible: how to stay vital, productive, and happy for a lifetime*. New York: McGraw-Hill Education.

Arias-Carrión, O., and E. Pöppel. 2007. "Dopamine, learning and reward-seeking behavior." *Acta Neurobiol Exp* 67 (4): 481-488.

Avena, Nicole M., Pedro Rada, and Bartley G. Hoebel. 2008. "Evidence for Sugar Addiction: Behavioral and Neurochemical Effects of Intermittent, Excessive Sugar Intake." *Neuroscience and Biobehavioral Reviews* 32 (1): 20-39. Accessed Jun 17, 2017.

Baumeister, et al. 1998. "Ego Depletion: Is the active self a limited resource?" *Journal of Personality and Social Psychology* 74 (5): 1252-1265.

Bentley, R., and R. Meganathan. 1982. "Biosynthesis of Vitamin K (menaquinone) in Bacteria." *Microbiological Reviews* 46 (3): 241-280.

Bernsmeier, A., and H. Hillesheim. 1958. "The glucose consumption of the brain & its dependence on the liver." *Arch Psychiatr Nervenkr Z Gesamte Neurol Psychiatr.* 196 (6): 611-626.

Berridge, K. C., T. E. Robinson, and J. W. Aldridge. 2009. "Dissecting components of reward: 'liking', 'wanting', and 'learning'." *Current Opinion in Pharmacology* 9 (1): 65-73. https://www.ncbi.nlm.nih.gov/pmc/articles/PMC2756052.

Besedovsky, H. O., A. Del Rey, and E. Sorkin. 1986. *Integration of Activated Immune Cell Products in Immune Endocrine Feedback Circuits.* Vol. 5, in *Leukocytes and Host Defense*, by J. J. Oppenheim and D. M. Jacobs, 200. New York: Alan R. Liss.

Brickman, P., D. Coates, and R. Janof-Bulman. 1978. "Lottery winners and accident victims: Is happiness relative?" *Journal of Personality and Social Psychology* 36 (8): 917-927.

Britta Hitze, et al. 2010. "How the Selfish Brain Organizes Its Supply and Demand." *Frontiers in Neuroenergetics* 2 (7). Accessed Jun 12, 2017.

Brown, R., and J. Kulik. 1977. "Flashbulb Memories." *Cognition* 5 (1): 73-99.

Bullemer, P., M. J. Nissen, and D. B. Willingham. 1989. "On the Development of Procedural Knowledge." *Journal of Experimental Psychology: Learning, Memory and Cognition* 15 (6): 1047-1060. doi:10.1037/0278-7393.15.6.1047.

Cacioppo, John T. et al. 2015. "The Neuroendocrinology of Social Isolation." *Annual Review of Psychology* 66: 733-767. Accessed Jun 17, 2017.

Cartee, Gregory D. et al. 2016. "Exercise Promotes Healthy Aging of Skeletal Muscle." *Cell Metabolism* 23 (6): 1034-1047. Accessed Jun 28, 2017.

Chiara, Gaetano di, and Assunta Imperato. 1988. "Drugs abused by humans preferentially increase synaptic dopamine concentrations in the mesolimbic system of freely moving rats." *National Academy of Sciences of the United States of America 84.* 5274-5278.

Christianson, S. A., and E. Loftus. 1990. "Some characteristics of people's traumatic memories."

Bulletin of the Psychonomic Society 28: 195-198. doi:10.3758/bf03334001.

Chyun, Y. S., B. E. Kream, and L. G. Raisz. 1984. "Cortisol decreases bone formation by inhibiting periosteal cell proliferation." *Endocrinology* 114 (2): 477-480. doi:10.1210/endo-114-2-477.

Coila, Bridgett. 2010. "Effects of Serotonin on the Body." *LiveStrong*. Jun 20. Accessed Aug 11, 2013. http://www.livestrong.com/article/154361-effects-of-serotonin-on-the-body/.

Colantuoni, C., J. Schwenker, J. McCarthy, P. Rada, B. Ladenheim, J. L. Cadet, G. J. Schwartz, T. H. Moran, and B. G. Hoebel. 2001. "Excessive sugar intake alters binding to dopamine and mu-opioid receptors in the brain." *Neuroreport* 12 (16): 3549-3552.

n.d. "Conscious parenting: parents as genetic engineers." *The biology of belief: unleashing the power of consciousness, matter & miracles*. 174.

Cottone, P., V. Savino, L. Steardo, and E. P. Zorrilla. 2008. "Opioid-dependent anticipatory negative contrast and binge-like eating in rats with limited access to highly preferred food." *Neuropsychopharmacology* 33 (3): 525-535.

Crone, Eveline. 2009. "Neurocognitive Development of Relational Reasoning." *Developmental Science* 12 (1): 55-66. Accessed Jul 6, 2017.

Cryan, J. F., and T. G. Dinan. 2012. "Mind-altering microorganisms: the impact of the gut microbiota on brain and behavior." *Nature Reviews Neuroscience* 3: 701-712.

Davidson, Richard. 2013. *The Emotional Life of Your Brain*. New York: Penguin Group.

Deci, E. L., and R. M. Ryan. 1985. *Intrinsic motivation and self-determination in human behavior*. New York: Plenum.

Deci, E. L., and R. M. Ryan. 2000. "The "What" And "Why" Of goal pursuits: Human needs and the self-determination of behavior." *Psychological Inquiry* 11: 227-268.

Deci, E. L., J. P. Connell, and R. M. Ryan. 1989. "Self-determination in a work organization." *Journal of Applied Psychology* 74: 580-590.

Desimone, R., and J. Duncan. 1995. "Neural mechanisms of selective visual attention." *Annu Rev Neurosci*, 193-222.

Despres, J. P. 2007. "Cardiovascular disease under the influence of excess visceral fat." *Crit Pathw Cardiol* 6 (2): 51-59. https://www.ncbi.nlm.nih.gov/pubmed/17667865.

DiChiara, G., and A. Imperato. 1988. "Drugs abused by humans preferentially increase synaptic dopamine concentrations in the mesolimbic system of freely moving rats." *Proc Natl Acad Sci USA* 85 (14): 5274-5278.

Dimitriadis, G., P. Mitrou, E. Maratou, and S. A. Raptis. 2011. "Insulin effects in muscle and adipose tissue."

Diabetes Research and Clinical Practice 93 (Suppl 1): S52-S59. https://www.researchgate.net/profile/Eirini_Maratou/publication/221930616_Insulin_effects_in_muscle_and_adipose_tissue/links/00b7d527a370a8fd76000000.pdf.

DiPellegrino, G., L. Fadiga, L. Fogassi, V. Gallese, and G. Rizzolatti. 1992. "Understanding Motor Events: A neurophysiological study." *Experimental Brain Research* 91: 176-180.

Dispenza, Joe. 2012. *Breaking the Habit of Being Yourself: How to Lose your Mind and Create a New One.* Carlsbad, CA: Hay House.

Dispenza, Joe, and Daniel G. Amen. 2015. "Survival vs. Creation." In *Breaking the habit of being yourself: How to lose your mind and create a new one*, 104-105. Carlsbad, CA: Hay House.

Doyle, John R. 2013. "Survey of time preference, delay discounting models"." *Judgment and Decision Making* 8 (2): 116-135. http://journal.sjdm.org/12/12309/jdm12309.pdf.

Drewnowski, A. 1998. "Energy density, palatability, and satiety: Implications for weight control." *Nutr Rev* 56: 347-353.

Drewnowski, A. 1997a. "Taste preferences and food intake." *Ann Rev Nutr* 17: 237-253.

Dudai, Y. 2004. "The Neurobiology of Consolidations, Or, How Stable is the Engram?" *Annual Review of Psychology* 55: 51-86. doi:10.1146/annurev. psych.55.090902.142050.

Duhigg, Charles. 2013. *The power of habit: why we do what we do in life and business.* Hà Nội: Lao động - Xã hội.

E. R. Sewell, et al. 2004. "Mapping Changes in the Human Cortex Throughout the Span of Life." *Neuroscientist* 10 (4): 372-392.

Encyclopaedia Britannica. 2011. "Blind Spot." http:// www.britannica.com/EBchecked/topic/69390/ blind-spot.

Eshak, E. S., H. Iso, C. Date, S. Kikuchi, Y. Watanabe, Y. Wada, K. Wakai, A. Tamakoshi, and JACC Study Group. 2010. "Dietary fiber intake is associated with reduced risk of mortality from cardiovascular disease among Japanese men and women." *J Nutr* 140 (8): 1445-1453.

Fehm, H. L., W. Kern, and A. Peters. 2006. "The selfish brain: competition for energy resources." *Progress in Brain Research* 153: 129-140.

Festinger, L. 1962. "Cognitivie Dissonance." *Scientific American* 207 (4): 93-107. doi:10.1038/ scientificamerican1062-93.

Feynman, Richard. 1970. *The Feynman Lectures on Physics Vol I.* Addison Wesley. http://www.feyn-manlectures.caltech.edu/I_04.html.

Floresco, S. B. n.d. "The Nucleus Accumbens: an interface between cognition, emotion, and action."

Annual Review of Psychology, 25-52. Accessed September 24, 2015. doi:10.1146/annurev-psych-010213-115159.pmid25251489.

Forcato, C. 2007. "Reconsolidation of Declarative Memory in Humans." *Learn Mem* 14 (4): 295-303.

Gailliot, M. T., R. F. Baumeister, C. N. DeWall, J. K. Maner, E. A. Plant, and D. M., et al. Tice. 2007. "Self-control relies on glucose as a limited energy source: Willpower is more than a metaphor." *Journal of Personality and Social Psychology* 92: 325-336.

Gladwell, Malcolm. 2008. *Outliers: the story of success.* New York: Back Bay, Little, Brown and Company.

Goodwin, M. L. 2010. "Blood Glucose Regulation during Prolonged, Submaximal, Continuous Exercise: A Guide for Clinicians." *Journal of Diabetes Science and Technology* 4 (3): 694-705.

Graybiel, Ann M. 2002. "Habits, Rituals, and the Evaluative Brain." *Annual Review of Neuroscience* 31: 1158-1161.

Graybiel, Ann M. 2005. "The Basal Ganglia: Learning New Tricks and Loving It." *Current Opinion in Neurobiology* 15: 638-44.

Hamann, S. B. 2001. "Cognitive and neural mechanisms of emotional memory." *Trends in Cognitive Sciences* 5 (9): 394-400. doi:10.1016/s1364-6613(00)01707-1.PMID11520704.

He, F. J., and G. A. MacGregor. 2007. "Salt, blood pressure and cardiovascular disease." *Curr Opin Cardiol.* 22 (4): 298-305.

Hebb, D. O. 1949. *The Organization of Behavior.* New York: Wiley & Sons.

Hoehn, K., and E. N. Marieb. 2010. *Human Anatomy & Physiology.* San Francisco: Benjamin Cummings.

Holland, Peter C. 1984. "Animal Behavior Processes." *Journal of Experimental Psychology* 10 (4): 461-475.

Hom, H. L., and R. A. Fabes. 1985. "The Role of Choice in Children's Ability to Delay Gratification." *Journal of Genetic Psychology* 146: 429-430.

Hu, Y., G. Block, E. P. Norkus, J. D. Morrow, M. Dietrich, and M. Hudes. 2006. "Relations of glycemic index and glycemic load with plasma oxidative stress markers." *Am J Clin Nutri* 84 (1): 70-6.

Hughes, John R. 1958. "Post-tetanic Potentiation." *Physiological Reviews* 38 (1): 91-113. doi:PMID13505117.

Hutchinson. 1965. "The Niche: an abstractly inhabited hypervolume." https://en.wikipedia.org/wiki/Adaptation#CITEREFHutchinson1965.

Indiana University (Department of Biology). n.d. *Biology of Food: The Bliss Point.* Accessed Apr 2, 2015. http://courses.bio.indiana.edu/L104-Bonner/F12/imagesF12/L8/BlissPoint.html.

Jansen, R. W., C. M. Connelly, M. M. Kelley-Gagnon, J. A. Parker, and L. A. Lipsitz. 1995. "Postprandial hypotension in elderly patients with unexplained syncope." *Arch Intern Med* 155 (9): 945-952.

K. J. Lee et al. 2013. "Motor Skill Training Induces Coordinated Strengthening and Weakening between Neighboring Synapses." *Journal of Neuroscience* 33 (23): 9794-9799.

K. Vohs, et al. 2011. "Ego depletion is not just fatigue: Evidence from a total sleep deprivation experiment." *Social Psychology and Personality Science* 18 (2): 166-173.

Keysers, Christian, and Valeria Gazzola. 2006. "Progress in Brain Research." Accessed Jun 30, 2007. https://web.archive.org/web/20070630021020/ .

Khurana. 2008. *Essentials of Medical Physiology*. Elsevier. https://books.google.ca/books?id=Cm_kLhU1AP0C&pg=PA460.

King, M. W. n.d. "The Medical Biochemistry Page." *Indiana University School of Medicine*. Accessed Dec 1, 2009. http://themedicalbiochemistrypage.org/nerves.html#5ht.

King, Wendy C., Jia-Yuh Chen, MS, and James E. et al. Mitchell, MD. 2012. "Prevalence of Alcohol Use Disorders Before and After Bariatric Surgery." *JAMA*, 2516-2525. doi:10.1001/jama.2012.6147.

Koestner, R., R. M. Ryan, F. Bernieri, and K. Holt. 1984. "Setting limits on children's behavior: The differential effects of controlling vs. Informational styles on intrinsic motivation and creativity." *Journal of Personality* 52: 233-248.

Kolb, Bryan, and Robbin Gibb. 2011. "Brain Plasticity and Behaviour in the Developing Brain." *Journal of the Canadian Academy of Child and Adolescent Psychiatry*, 265-276.

Krieger, M. 1921. "On the atrophy on human organs in inanition." *Z. Angew Anat. Konstitutionsl.* 7: 87-134.

LaBar, K. S., and R. Cabeza. 2006. "Cognitive Neuroscience of Emotional Memory." *Nature Rev Neuro* 7: 54-64.

Lattimer, James M., and Mark D. Haub. 2010. "Effects of Dietary Fiber and Its Components on Metabolic Health." *Nutrients* 2 (12): 1266-1289. Accessed Jun 17, 2017.

Lazarus, R. S. 1991. *Emotion and Adaptation*. New York: Oxford University Press.

Lee, Mary R. 2016. "Targeting the Oxytocin System to Treat Addictive Disorders: Rationale and Progress to Date." *CNS Drugs* 30 (2): 109-123. Accessed Jun 17, 2017.

Lehrer, Jonah. 2009. "Don't!: The Secret of Self Control." *The New Yorker*. http://www.newyorker.com/reporting/2009/05/18/090518fa_fact_lehrer.

Levenson, R. W. 1994. "Human emotions: A functional view." In *The Nature of Emotion: Fundamental questions*, edited by P. Ekman and R. Davidson, 123-126. New York: Oxford University Press.

Linus Pauling Institute. 2014. *Micronutrient Information Center*. Corvallis, OR, Jul. Accessed Mar 20, 2017.

Lipton, Bruce H. 2016. "Conscious Parenting." In *The biology of belief: unleashing the power of consciousness, matter & miracles*, 176-178. Carlsbad, CA: Hay House, Inc.

Livingston, M., and D. Hubel. 1988. "Segregation of Form, Colour, Movement and Depth: Anatomy, Physiology and Perception." *Science* 240: 740-749.

Logothetis, N. K. 1998. "Single Units and Conscious Vision." *Philosophical Transactions of the Royal Society B: Biological Sciences*, 1801-1818.

Logothetis, N. K., and D. L. Sheinberg. 1996. "Visual object recognition." *Annu Rev Neurosci* 19: 577-621.

Lowette, Katrien et al. 2015. "Effects of High-Fructose Diets on Central Appetite Signaling and Cognitive Function." *Frontiers in Nutrition* 2: 5. Accessed Jun 17, 2017.

M. Muraven, et al. 2008. "Helpful self-control: Autonomy support, vitality, and depletion." *Journal of Experimental Social Psychology* 44 (3): 573-585.

Ma, Xiao et al. 2017. "The Effect of Diaphragmatic Breathing on Attention, Negative Affect and Stress in Healthy Adults." *Frontiers in Psychology* 8: 874. Accessed Jul 6, 2017.

Mackay, D. G., M. Shafto, J. K. Taylor, D. E. Marian, L. Abrams, and J. R. Dyer. 2004. "Relations between emotion, memory, and attention: Evidence from taboo Stroop, lexical decision, and immediate memory tasks." *Memory & Cognition* 32 (3): 474-488.

Malenka, R. C., E. J. Nestler, and S. E. Hyman. 2009. "Molecular Neuropharmacology: A Foundation for Clinical Neuroscience." Edited by A. Sydor and R. Y. Brown, 147-148, 366-367, 375-376. New York: McGraw-Hill Medical.

Mather, George. n.d. "The Visual Cortex." *School of Life Sciences: University of Sussex.* Accessed Mar 6, 2017. http://www.lifesci.sussex.ac.uk/home/George_Mather/Linked Pages/Physiol/Cortex.html.

Mathes, Wendy Foulds et al. 2009. "The Biology of Binge Eating." *Appetite* 52 (3): 545-553. Accessed Jun 17, 2017.

Maton, Anthea, Jean Hopkins, Charles William McLaughlin, Susan Johnson, Maryanna Quon Warner, David LaHart, and Jill D. Wright. 1993. *Human Biology and Health.* Englewood Cliffs, NJ: Prentice Hall.

Mayer, F. L., D. Wilson, and B. Hube. 2013. *Virulence* 4: 119-128.

McCorry, Laurie Kelly. 2007. "Physiology of the Autonomic Nervous System." *American Journal of Pharmaceutical Education* 71 (4): 78.

McGuire, Michael. 2013. *Believing, the neuroscience of fantasies, fears and confictions*. Prometius Books.

Metcalfe, J., and A. P. Shimamura. 1994. *Metacognition: knowing about knowing*. Cambridge, MA: MIT Press.

Miller, A. K. H., R. L. Alston, and J. A. N. Corsellis. 1980. "Variation with Age in the Volumes of Grey and White Matter in the Cerebral Hemispheres of Man: Measurements with an Image Analyser." *Neuropathology and Applied Neurobiology* 6 (2): 119-132.

Mischel, Walter, Yuichi Shoda, and Monica L. Rodriguez. 1989. "Delay of gratification in children." *Science* 244: 933-938. doi:10.1126/science.2658056.

Muraven, M., and R. Baumeister. 2000. "Self-regulation and depletion of limited resources: Does self-control resemble a muscle?" *Psychological Bulletin* 126 (2): 247-259.

Muraven, M., R. L. Collins, and K. Nienhaus. 2002. "Self-control and alcohol restraint: An initial application of the self-control strength model." *Psychology of Addictive Behaviors* 16: 113-120.

National Institute of Diabetes and Digestive and Kidney Diseases. 2008. "Hypoglycemia." Oct. Accessed Jun 28, 2015.

Nehlig, Astrid. 2013. "The Neuroprotective Effects of Cocoa Flavanol and Its Influence on Cognitive Performance." *British Journal of Clinical*

Pharmacology 75 (3): 716-727. Accessed Jun 17, 2017.

Nieoullon, A., and A. Coquere. 2003. "Dopamine: A Key Regulator to Adapt Action, Emotion, Motivation and Cognition." *Curr Opin Neurol Suppl* 2: S3-S9.

Nowak, Jan K. et al. 2014. "Prevalence and Correlates of Vitamin K Deficiency in Children with Inflammatory Bowel Disease." *Scientific Reports* 4: 4768. Accessed Jun 17, 2017.

Offer, D. et al. 2000. "The Altering of Reported Experiences." *J. of Child & Adol Psych* 33 (6): 735-742.

Ogden, C. L., S. Z. Yanovski, M. D. Carroll, and K. M. Flegal. 2007. "The Epidemiology of Obesity." *Gastroenterology* 2087-2102.

Öhman, A. 2000. "Fear and anxiety: Evolutionary, cognitive, and clinical perspectives." In *Handbook of Emotions*, edited by M. Lewis and J. M. Haviland-Jones, 573-593. New York: The Guilford Press.

2016. "Pattern Recognition and Your Brain." *Psychology24.org*. Mar 21. Accessed May 23, 2017. http://www.psychology24.org/pattern-recognition-and-your-brain/.

Pickles, James O. 2012. *An Introduction to the Physiology of Hearing*. 4th. Bingley: Emerald Group Publishing Limited.

Quigley, Eamonn M. M. 2013. "Gut Bacteria in Health and Disease." *Gastroenterology & Hepatology* 9 (9): 560-569.

Quiroga, Rodrigo Quian, and Carlos Pedreira. 2011. "How Do We See Art: An Eye-Tracker Study." *Frontiers in Human Neuroscience* 5: 98. Accessed Jun 18, 2017.

2015. "Relaxation techniques: Breath control helps quell errant stress response." *Harvard Health Publications, Harvard Medical School.* Jan. Accessed Sep 11, 2017. http://www.health.harvard.edu/mind-and-mood/relaxation-techniques-breath-control-helps-quell-errant-stress-response.

Rizzolatti, Giacomo, Luciano Fadiga, Vittorio Gallese, and Leonardo Fogassi. 1996. "Premotor cortex and the recognition of motor actions." *Cognitive Brain Research* 3 (2): 131-141. https://www.researchgate.net/publication/14487934.

Rosenzweig, M. R. 1996. "Aspects of the Search for Neural Mechanisms of Memory." *Annual Review of Psychology* 47: 1-32.

Ross, M. 1989. "Relation of implicit theories to the construction of personal histories." *Psychological Review* 96: 341-357.

Satija, A., and F. B. Hu. 2012. "Cardiovascular benefits of dietary fiber." *Curr Atheroscler Rep* 14 (6): 505-514.

Saulnier, Delphine M. et al. 2013. "The Intestinal Microbiome, Probiotics and Prebiotics in Neurogastroenterology." *Gut Microbes* 4 (1): 17-27. Accessed Jun 17, 2017.

Schacter, D. L. 1987. "Implicit Memory: History and current status." *Journal of Experimental Psychology: Learning, Memory, and Cognition* 13: 501-518. doi:10.1037/0278-7393.13.3.501.

Seifert, T., P. Brassard, M. Wissenberg, P. Rasmussen, P. Nordby, B. Stallknecht, H. Adser, A. H. Jakobsen, H. Pilegaard, and H. B. Nielsen et al. 2010. "Endurance training enhances BDNF release from the human brain." *Am J Physiol Regul Integr Comp Physiol* 298 (2): R372-377.

Shirey, L. L. 1992. "Importance, Interest and Selective Attention." In *The Role of Interest in Learning and Development*, edited by K. A. Renninger et al., 281-296. Hillsdale, NJ: Lawrence Erlbaum Assoc.

Singh, Minati. 2014. "Mood, Food, and Obesity." *Frontiers in Psychology* 5: 925. Accessed Jun 17, 2017.

Stahl, S. M., L. Mignon, and J. M. Meyer. 2009. "Which comes first: atypical antipsychotic treatment or cardiometabolic risk?" *Acta Psychiatr Scand* 119 (3): 171-179.

Stanhope, Kimber L. 2016. "Sugar Consumption, Metabolic Disease and Obesity: The State of the Controversy." *Critical Reviews in Clinical*

Laboratory Sciences 53 (1): 52-67. Accessed Jun 17, 2017.

Starr, Cecie. 2005. *Biology: Concepts and Applications*. Thomas Brooks/Cole. https://books.google.com/?id=RtSpGV_Pl_0C&pg=PA94.

Steimer, Thierry. 2002. "The Biology of Fear- and Anxiety-Related Behaviors." *Dialogues in Clinical Neuroscience* 4 (3): 231-249.

2016. "The Asch Experiment: The Power of Peer Pressure." *Boundless*. May 26. Accessed Jan 14, 2017. https://www.boundless.com/sociology/textbooks/boundless-sociology-textbook/social-groups-and-organization-6/group-dynamics-57/the-asch-experiment-the-power-of-peer-pressure-356-3293/.

Théoret, Hugo, and Alvaro Pascual-Leone. 2002. "Language Acquisition: Do as You Hear." *Current Biology* 12 (21): R736-R737.

Tice, D. M., R. F. Baumeister, D. Shmueli, and M. Muraven. 2007. "Restoring the self: Positive affect helps improve self-regulation following ego depletion." *Journal of Experimental Social Psychology* 43: 379-384.

Tooby, J., and L. Cosmides. 1990. "The past explains the present: Emotional adaptations and the structure of ancestral environments." *Ethology and Sociobiology* 11: 375-424.

Trifilieff, Pierre, and Diana Martinez. 2014. "Imaging Addiction: D2 Receptors and Dopamine Signaling in the Striatum as Biomarkers for Impulsivity." *Neuropharmacology* 76: 498-509. Accessed Jun 18, 2017.

Turnbaugh, P. J. et al. 2006. "An obesity-associated gut microbiome with increased capacity for energy harvest." *Nature* 444: 1027-1031.

Vickers, Andrew, Catherine Zollman, and David K. Payne. 2001. "Hypnosis and Relaxation Therapies." *Western Journal of Medicine* 175 (4): 269-272.

Vohs, K., et al. 2005. "Self-regulation and self-presentation: Regulatory resource depletion impairs impression management and effortful self-presentation depletes regulatory resources." *Journal of Personality and Social Psychology* 88 (4): 632-657.

Weindruch, R., and R. S. Sohal. 1997. "Seminars in medicine of the Beth Israel Deaconess Medical Center. Caloric intake and aging." *New England Journal of Medicine* 337 (14): 986-994.

Wildt, Grace. n.d. "The Bliss Point." *Retro Report.* Accessed Jan 6, 2016. http://www.retroreport.org/voices/the-bliss-point/.

Williams, G. C., V. M. Grow, Z. R. Freedman, R. M. Ryan, and E. L. Deci. 1996. "Motivational predictors of weight loss and weight-loss maintenance." *Journal of Personality and Social Psychology* 70: 115-126.

Williams, Kristine, and Susan Kemper. 2010. "Exploring Interventions to Reduce Cognitive Decline in Aging." *Journal of Psychosocial Nursing and Mental Health Services* 48 (5): 42-51. Accessed Jun 17, 2017.

Woods, Stephen C. 2004. "Gastrointestinal Satiety Signals I: An overview of gastrointestinal signals that influence food intake." *Journal of Physiology: Gastrointestinal and Liver Physiology* 286 (1): G7-13.

Wu, J., H. Xiao, H. Sun, L. Zou, and L. Q. Zhu. 2012. "Role of Dopamine Receptors in ADHD: a systematic meta-analysis." 45 (3): 605-620. doi:10.1007/s12035-012-8278-5.PMID22610946.

Yang, H. P., L. Wang, L. Han, and S. C. Wang. 2013. "Nonsocial functions of hypothalamic oxytocin." *ISRN Neuroscience* 179-272. https://www.ncbi.nlm.nih.gov/pmc/articles/PMC4045544.

Yang, Y., and A. Raine. 2009. "Prefrontal structural and functional brain imaging findings in antisocial, violent, and psychopathic individuals: a meta-analysis." *Psychiatry Research* 174 (2): 81-88. https://www.ncbi.nlm.nih.gov/pmc/articles/PMC2784035.

Recommended Readings

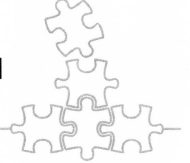

BREAKING THE HABIT OF BEING YOURSELF: How to Lose Your Mind and Create a New One,
by Dr. Joe Dispenza

THE BIOLOGY OF BELIEF: Unleashing the Power of Consciousness, Matter & Miracles,
by Dr. Bruce H. Lipton

THE BIOLOGY OF DESIRE: Why Addiction is Not a Disease, by Marc Lewis

THE BREAKTHROUGH EXPERIENCE: A Revolutionary New Approach to Personal Transformation, by Dr. John Demartini

THE ANATOMY OF THE SPIRIT: The Seven Stages of Power and Healing, by Dr. Caroline Myss

THE POWER OF HABIT: Why We Do What We do, and How to Change, by Charles Duhigg

Index

abdominal breathing, 173
adrenaline 87, 125, 161,
advertisement 5, 10,
aerobic exercise *see* also physical exercise 86, 123
amygdala 123-124, 163, 172, 178,
anticipation 104, 135
anxiety 71, 95, 115, 148-153, 162, 172
appetite xii, 11, 53, 60, 66, 70, 80, 84, 91, 159
autopilot *see* also default mode network (DMN) 6, 119, 140

bacteria 68-72
    candida 72-73
blood brain barrier 58
blood sugar 37, 54-57, 61-64, 93, 124-125, 161
brain-derived neurotrophic factor (BDNF) 86, 123
brain-wave(s) 184-185
    Beta 184

    Alpha 184-185
    Delta 185
    Theta 184-185
breakfast 55, 62

caffeine 59, 61
calories 66, 92, 95, 96, 125
carbohydrate 54, 55, 59, 61, 62, 63, 93
cheat day(s) 89-91
chewing 63, 87
chocolate xiv, 10, 26, 64-66, 83-84, 95
cognitive dissonance 136-137, 177
cognitive empathy 78
consolidation 106
core need *see* also reward 142
cortisol 87, 161
cravings 10, 55-59, 61, 64, 66, 71-72, 105, 137, 141-142, 181
cue 4-5, 7, 9-19, 24, 62-63, 105, 119, 135, 143, 193,

Endnotes

1   These figures come from four graphs that compare the response of four drugs and the dopamine they release. See Gaetano di Chiara and Assunta Imperato, "Drugs abused by humans preferentially increase synaptic dopamine concentrations in the mesolimbic system of freely moving rats" Proceedings of the National Academy of Sciences of the United States of America 84, no. 14 (July 1988): 5274-78.

CPSIA information can be obtained
at www.ICGtesting.com
Printed in the USA
LVOW12s0455281117
557835LV00001B/29/P